CBT for Chronic Pain and Psychologi

CBT for Chronic Pain and Psychological Well-Being

A Skills Training Manual Integrating DBT, ACT, Behavioral Activation and Motivational Interviewing

Dr. Mark Carlson

WILEY Blackwell

This edition first published 2014
© 2014 John Wiley & Sons, Ltd.

Registered Office
John Wiley & Sons Ltd, The Atrium, Southern Gate, Chichester, West Sussex, PO19 8SQ, UK

Editorial Offices
350 Main Street, Malden, MA 02148-5020, USA

9600 Garsington Road, Oxford, OX4 2DQ, UK

The Atrium, Southern Gate, Chichester, West Sussex, PO19 8SQ, UK

For details of our global editorial offices, for customer services, and for information about how to apply for permission to reuse the copyright material in this book please see our website at www.wiley.com/wiley-blackwell.

The right of Mark Carlson to be identified as the author of this work has been asserted in accordance with the UK Copyright, Designs and Patents Act 1988.

Library of Congress Cataloging-in-Publication Data
Carlson, Mark (Mark Stanley), 1952– author.
    CBT for chronic pain and psychological well-being: a skills training manual integrating DBT, ACT, behavioral activation and motivational interviewing / Mark Carlson.
        pages cm
    Includes bibliographical references and index.
    ISBN 978-1-118-78881-3 (paperback)
    1. Chronic pain–Treatment. 2. Cognitive therapy. 3. Evidence-based psychotherapy. I. Title.
RB127.C377 2014
616.89'0472–dc23
                            2013050479

A catalogue record for this book is available from the British Library.

Cover image: © Cosmo Condina/Getty Images

Set in 10/12.5 pt on GalliardStd-Roman by Toppan Best-set Premedia Limited

1 2014

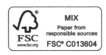

Contents

To:

Jules and Spencer – I love you both with all of my heart

Mom and Dad – your love and support means the world to me

Grandma and Grandpa – I wish you would have been able to stay with us longer

Acknowledgments

I would like to thank all of the people at Wiley Blackwell who made this project complete. Fiona, Allison, Karen, Darren and Andrew – you have all been great to work with!

Special acknowledgment goes to the "pain team" at Mental Health Systems (MHS):

Brittany Holtberg – great work and thanks for all that you have done.
Morgan Cusack, Meagan Karsten, and Amy Gimbel – I could not have asked for better clinicians to work with.
Dr. Chris Malone – you were a great help throughout the process.
Dave Karan and Krista Peterson – thanks for your contributions to the process.
Lane, Steve, Shelley, and Michael – I could not have done this without your support and friendship.

Chapter 1

Introduction to Comorbid Mental Health and Chronic Pain

The prevalence and cost of chronic pain is a growing concern in the United States. During the past decade, increasing research focus on exploring treatment for chronic pain has led to important implications for current coordination of medical and psychological management to treat individuals suffering with chronic pain. There are relatively few research articles that are not diagnosis- or syndrome-specific, with even fewer random clinical trials (RCTs) or meta-analytic studies. In their research, Elliott and colleagues (1999) have indicated that at least 45 percent of Americans will seek treatment or care for chronic pain at some point in their lives, making a total of over 50 million people in the United States. The Centers for Disease Control and Prevention reported that in 2005, 133 million Americans were experiencing chronic illness, equivalent to almost 1 out of every 2 adults. Nearly a quarter of people with chronic conditions also reported experiencing limitations to daily activity due to their illness, and also experienced clinical mental health concerns. Currently, children suffering from chronic illnesses that were considered fatal in the past now live well into adulthood, thanks to advances in medical care. While these advances are promising, they can result in prolonged lifespans and chronic pain (Martinez, 2009). In response to such findings, in 2010 the Joint Commission on Accreditation of Healthcare Organizations established a requirement for physicians to consider pain as a fifth vital sign, in addition to pulse, blood pressure, core temperature, and respiration (Gatchel, Peng, Peters, Fuchs, & Turk, 2007). Survival from chronic health conditions brings new challenges for individuals throughout their lifespan, including physical, psychological and social adjustment difficulties.

Health Care Costs

Chronic pain is associated with a wide range of illness, injury, disease, and mental health issues, and it is sometimes the primary concern in and of itself. With some

CBT for Chronic Pain and Psychological Well-Being: A Skills Training Manual Integrating DBT, ACT, Behavioral Activation and Motivational Interviewing, First Edition. Mark Carlson.
© 2014 John Wiley & Sons, Ltd. Published 2014 by John Wiley & Sons, Ltd.

conditions, pain and the associated symptoms arise from a discrete cause, such as postoperative pain or pain associated with a malignancy. In other situations pain constitutes the primary problem, such as neuropathic pains or headaches. Millions suffer from acute or chronic pain every year and the effects of pain take a tremendous toll on our country in terms of health care costs, rehabilitation, and lost worker productivity, as well as in terms of the emotional and financial burden placed on patients and their families. The costs of pain can result in longer hospital stays, higher rates of re-hospitalization, more emergency room visits, more unnecessary medical visits, and a reduced ability to function that leads to lost income and insurance coverage. As such, patients' unrelieved chronic pain often results in an inability to work and maintain health insurance.

According to a recent Institute of Medicine Report titled *Relieving Pain in America: A Blueprint for Transforming Prevention, Care, Education, and Research*, pain is a significant public health problem that costs society at least $560–$635 billion annually, an amount equal to about $2,000 for every person living in the United States. This includes the total incremental cost of health care due to pain ranging from $261 to $300 billion, and losses of productivity and associated issues ranging from $297–$336 billion.

Chronic Pain and Function

Pain is a complex sensational experience resulting from brain signals and damage or irritations to the nervous system, and is encompassed by cognitions, sensory-motor input, emotions, and hormone systems (Gatchel, 2004). Pain can be caused by chronic medical conditions, neuropathic trauma, injury, and accidents (American Society of Anesthesiologists, 2010). Acute pain is short term and temporary. Chronic pain is long term with symptoms exceeding three months (Lewandowski, 2006). The comorbidity of mental health and physical problems resulting from pain is well established in the research (Gatchel, 2004). Common comorbidity includes anxiety, depression, adjustment disorder, obsessive-compulsive disorder (OCD), histrionic personality disorder, and borderline personality disorder (BPD). The trigger is the pain and uncertain prognosis of the diagnosed condition, specifically around progression of the disease, recurrence, reduced lifespan, end-of-life issues, treatment and side-effects, cognitive, physical, and behavioral impairments, and functional limitations (Ownsworth, 2009). Pain often results from chronic illness, injury, degeneration, and many related triggers in a chronic population. People who experience chronic pain often experience a decrease in quality of life including: overall physical and emotional health; psychological and social well-being; fulfillment of personal expectations and goals; economic burden and financial stability; functional capacity to carry out daily routines; and activities of daily living. Additionally, destruction of family and social life, problems with treatment adherence and support systems, and decreased participation in sports or leisure activities have been found to increase the risk of clinical anxiety and depression, resulting in greater functional impairment and poor quality of life (Gatchel *et al.*, 2007). This functional impairment and reduction in quality of life often leads to a variety of mental health concerns including demoralization and a reduction in effective participation in treatment as well as life in general.

Medical Interventions

There are a variety of medical interventions that are frequently implemented in the treatment of chronic pain. The American Society of Anesthesiologists Task Force (2010) conducted a literature review of treatment techniques for chronic pain and noted research support for the following nine interventions: ablative techniques, acupuncture, blocks (e.g., joint and nerve or nerve root), botulinum toxin injections, electrical nerve stimulation, epidural steroids with or without local anesthetics, intrathecal drug therapies, minimally invasive spinal procedures, and trigger point injections. The recommendations for use vary depending on the epidemiology of the chronic pain condition in question.

Pharmacotherapy

Pharmacologic management is often included in the treatment regimen of chronic pain conditions. Pharmacotherapy for the treatment of chronic pain includes the use of anticonvulsants, antidepressants, benzodiazepines, *N*-methyl-D-aspartate (NDMA) receptor antagonists, nonsteriodal antiiflammatory drugs (NSAIDs), opioid therapy (e.g., oral, transdermal, transmucosal, internasal, and sublingual), skeletal muscle relaxants, and topical agents (American Society of Anesthesiologists, 2010).

Physical therapy

The use of physical or restorative therapies for the treatment of chronic pain, particularly with back pain, has also been popular. A review of available research on the use of physical or restorative therapies for the treatment of chronic pain conducted by the American Society of Anesthesiologists (2010) indicated promising results. Randomized controlled trials that incorporated a variety of these therapies, such as with fitness classes, exercise therapy, and physiotherapy, were effective for treating low back pain. American Society of Anesthesiologists and American Society of Regional Anesthesia members recommended that physical or restorative therapies be implemented in the treatment strategy for patients with low back pain, as well as for other chronic pain conditions.

Cognitive Behavioral Therapy

Cognitive factors play an important role in the experience of chronic pain (Gatchel *et al.*, 2007). Cognitive Behavioral Therapy (CBT) interventions are based on the view that an individual's beliefs, evaluation, and interpretation about his or her health condition, in addition to pain, disability, and coping abilities, will impact the degree of both physical and emotional disability of the pain condition. CBT-based techniques currently vary widely in the literature, and can include distraction, imagery, motivational self-talk, relaxation training, biofeedback, development of coping strategies, goal setting, and changing maladaptive beliefs about pain.

Morely, Eccleston, and Williams (1999) conducted a meta-analysis of randomized trials of Cognitive Behavioral Therapy (CBT) for treating clients with chronic pain. Their findings concluded that the use of CBT treatment to replace maladaptive patient cognitions and behaviors with more adaptive ones is effective for a variety of pain conditions. More recently, Linton and Nordin (2006) reported a 5-year follow-up of a randomized controlled trial of CBT intervention for clients suffering from chronic back pain. Their results indicated that CBT interventions (compared to the control group) resulted in significantly less pain, a more active life, higher perceived quality of life, and better overall health. In addition, significant economic benefits were associated with the clients who had completed CBT treatment.

Multimodal interventions

Multimodal interventions include the use of more than one type of therapy for the treatment of patients with chronic pain. Multidisciplinary interventions bring together multimodality approaches within the context of a treatment program that consists of more than one discipline. After a review of the literature on the treatment of chronic pain, the American Society of Anesthesiologists Task Force on Chronic Pain Management (2010) concluded that in comparison to conventional treatment programs, multidisciplinary treatment programs are more effective in reducing the intensity of pain reported by patients with chronic pain. Based on the research, the Task Force recommends that multimodal interventions should be part of the treatment plan for patients with chronic pain, and implemented within multidisciplinary teams if available.

Current psychological treatment modalities and levels of care

There currently appear to be three levels of care for clients suffering from chronic pain in the United States. The first level of care is primary medical treatment. This tends to be carried out in hospitals and interventions are based upon medical treatments for pain. This level involves assessment, surgery, acute-care, recovery, and is staffed primarily with medical teams and supplementary work with physical therapists and occupational therapists. Psychological interventions at this level typically operate in more of an ancillary fashion, and include assessment and interventions designed to assist the individual with planned medical procedures. The second level of care is more diverse in service options. At this level of care, hospitals, emergency rooms, outpatient medical programs, and specialty pain programs typically provide treatment. Psychological interventions at this level typically include time-limited individual therapy, biofeedback training, supportive group work, and psychoeducation to families and clients. Many pain programs incorporate psychological work at this level through ancillary treatment or manualized program options designed to support the work of the medical interventions. Research does not indicate any standard manualized approach that is either accepted or used across programs. Inpatient programs and specialty pain programs appear to have their own psychological treatment manuals and standards of care for clients, but the content varies to a great degree. Some distinct commonalities are found, however: cognitive behavioral work with clients, relaxation training, biofeedback, and a growing emphasis on mindfulness. The third level of care is general outpatient work with clients. This level may include working with medical teams, rehabilitation and restorative therapies, work force training, and potentially worker's compensation claims. The client may have exhausted medical interventions and be faced with learning to accept their status and changes in functioning and quality of life. Psychological interventions at this level tend to include individual therapy, biofeedback training, supportive group work, and psychoeducation to clients and families.

It is clear that the medical model is the primary intervention strategy for levels one and two. Psychological interventions are typically considered to be supportive and ancillary in nature. When faced with the reality of having pain be a part of their lives with little or no hope for positive change or a cure, demoralization is a common reaction for many clients. The field of psychology has few treatment manuals and integrated treatment options for clients as they move to the third level of care. It is also quite clear that a client with comorbid mental health, chronic pain, and chemical use problems has few if any integrated treatment options available to them. This manual aims to provide practitioners with one of the first comprehensive guides to treating clients at levels two and three – and which can be applied across modalities and multiple levels of care.

Chapter 2

Treatment Organization, Outline, and Structure of the Program

The TAG (Teach, Apply, and Generalize) program has its roots in the philosophy of contextualism. Leaders in the philosophy of contextualism include James, Dewey, Mead, K. Burke, and Bormann. The predominant character of behavior analysis or at least what is central and distinctive about behavior analysis, is contextualistic (Hayes 1988). The philosophy of contextualism corresponds well with Behavioral Analytic concepts of the operant, accomplishment of attainable goals, the active role of the therapist, and working with order and randomness. The TAG program incorporates these key concepts into its fundamental structure and operations. The TAG program is based on Cognitive Behavioral Therapy through practice, primary intervention strategies, and skills training. The TAG program incorporates skills and concepts from: Dialectical Behavior Therapy (DBT), Motivational Interviewing (MI), Acceptance and Commitment Therapy (ACT), and Behavioral Activation (BA). The TAG curriculum also includes grief and loss work, Existential approaches, relapse-prevention, Mindfulness, identity development, and an additional track of service for individuals with substance dependence through DBT-S (dialectical behavior therapy for substance use disorders).

There are many theories and approaches in the field of psychology. Empirically Supported Treatments (ESTs) were identified and relevant research was reviewed in order to create the TAG program. It was decided to continue the development through a contextual model that incorporates components shared by all approaches to psychotherapy, as well as six elements that are common to the rituals and procedures used by all psychotherapists (see below). As Arkowitz (1992) reports, dissatisfaction with individual theoretical approaches spawned three movements: (a) theoretical integration, (b) technical eclecticism, and (c) common factors. The contextual model is a derivative of the common factors view (Wampold 2001).

According to Wampold (2001):

CBT for Chronic Pain and Psychological Well-Being: A Skills Training Manual Integrating DBT, ACT, Behavioral Activation and Motivational Interviewing, First Edition. Mark Carlson.
© 2014 John Wiley & Sons, Ltd. Published 2014 by John Wiley & Sons, Ltd.

A contextual model was proposed by Jerome Frank in his book, *Persuasion and Healing* (Frank & Frank 1991). According to Frank and Frank (1991), "the aim of psychotherapy is to help people feel and function better by encouraging appropriate modifications in their assumptive worlds, thereby transforming the meanings of experiences to more favorable ones" (p. 30). Persons who present for psychotherapy are demoralized and have a variety of problems, typically depression and anxiety. That is, people seek psychotherapy for the demoralization that results from their symptoms rather than from symptom relief. Frank has proposed that "psychotherapy achieves its effects largely and directly by treating demoralization and only indirectly treating overt symptoms of covert psychopathology" (Parloff, 1986, p. 522)

Frank and Frank (1991) described the components shared by all approaches to psychotherapy. The first component is that psychotherapy involves an emotionally charged, confiding relationship with a helping person (i.e., the therapist). The second component is that the context of the relationship is a healing setting, in which the client presents to a professional whom the client believes can provide help and who is entrusted to work in his or her behalf. The third component is that there exists a rationale, conceptual scheme, or myth that provides a plausible explanation for the patient's symptoms and prescribes a ritual or procedure for resolving them. The final component is a ritual or procedure that requires the active participation of both client and therapist and is based on the rationale (i.e., the ritual or procedure is believed to be a viable means of helping the client).

Frank and Frank (1991) discussed six elements that are common to the rituals and procedures used by all psychotherapists. First, the therapist combats the client's sense of alienation by developing a relationship that is maintained after the client divulges feelings of demoralization. Second, the therapist maintains the patient's expectation of being helped by linking hope for improvement to the process of therapy. Third, the therapist provides new learning experiences. Fourth, the client's emotions are aroused as a result of the therapy. Fifth, the therapist enhances the client's sense of mastery or self-efficacy. Sixth, the therapist provides opportunities for practice.

Wampold (2001) furthers this concept by adding that in the contextual model, specific ingredients are necessary to construct a coherent treatment that therapists have faith in and that provides a convincing rationale to clients.

The TAG program was created for individuals experiencing issues with comorbid mental health and chronic pain. The model that was adopted as a framework of understanding and organization is the biopsychosocial model of pain pioneered by G. L. Engel (1977).

According to Lewandowski (2006):

We are beginning to live in the era of the biopsychosocial (BPS) view of pain, which takes into account the biological (physical) influences, but also looks at the psychological (emotional) influences and places them in a social (personal) context.

The Cartesian (biological) model of pain

The explanation for pain that has dominated much of medical history came from the sixteenth-century Western philosopher, physiologist, and mathematician René

Descartes. The Cartesian model – essentially a biological model – set forth that anything that could be doubted should be rejected. Under Cartesian thinking, the only useful factor in the pain experience was tissue injury. Tissue injury could be measured; it could be proven. The degree of pain was assumed to be determined by and directly proportional to the degree of injury. Only the physical aspects of pain mattered. Any person with a particular injury was expected to feel and respond in exactly the same way as any other person with that same injury. In the Cartesian model, tissue injury can be likened to a dial controlling volume; turn up the injury, the tissue damage, and you turn up the pain. But chronic pain has been shown to be much less mechanistic.

The gate-control model of pain

The Cartesian theory was the firmly accepted way of looking at pain until 1965, when Ronald Melzack, a Canadian psychologist, and Patrick Wall, a British physiologist, put forth the gate-control theory of pain. Melzack and Wall (1988) argued that pain signals do not travel simply from the injured tissue to the brain; rather, those signals must go through a gating mechanism in the spinal cord. When the gate is closed, pain is not registered in the brain. When the gate is opened, pain registers. And the gate can be opened or closed by more factors than the signals caused by tissue damage.

The gate-control theory goes beyond a simple focus on the body and takes into account the impact of the mind. Melzack and Wall said that the gate could be opened or closed by emotions, memories, mood, and thoughts. After the signals reach a certain threshold, the brain generates pain sensations. In fact, the brain can register pain even when there is no tissue damage whatsoever (as with phantom pain from amputated limbs). PET scans have shown that parts of the brain light up with pain even when there is no tissue damage.

Despite wide acceptance of the gate-control theory of pain, today's physicians still tend to see pain in Cartesian terms (as a physical process and a sign of tissue damage) because they are trained in Cartesian terms. They know how to look for ruptured disks, fractures, infection, and disease. But when it comes to pain, most physicians get only a few hours of training in pain management, if they get any at all.

The biopsychosocial model: The future of pain management

While there are people who still believe that pain must not be real if a physical cause can't be found, the tide is turning. Unfortunately, some of the people questioning the reality of pain are medical professionals. But the more comprehensive and inclusive biopsychosocial model, pioneered by G. L. Engel (1977), is gaining widespread acceptance as more and more success is reported in its use.

One major drawback to the biological model was that it expected every person with the same injury to experience the same pain. There is no question that the focus of medicine on biological factors improved the quality of our lives. Take medications, for example. Antibiotics give us a powerful weapon against bacterial infections, anti-inflammatory medications reduce swelling and pain, and anti-hypertensives lower blood pressure. But the biological model did not consider external influences as relevant to disease in general and pain in particular.

Today, our understanding of pain has evolved and broadened. We are beginning to live in the era of the biopsychosocial (BPS) view of pain, which takes into account the biological (physical) influences but also looks at the psychological (emotional) influences and places them in a social (personal) context. The BPS model considers the entire person – body, mind, and environment.

The TAG Program for Chronic Pain and Psychological Well-Being – Structure, Purpose, and Rationale

The TAG program is designed to be 3–6+ months in duration and have flexibility in implementation across modalities of treatment. The concepts and skills training of the TAG program can be easily applied in individual therapy if that is the primary modality for intervention. The individual therapist will be able to modify the format and select concepts and skill sets to customize for the individual. This modification relies on the education, training, and expertise of the clinician since it deviates from the initial design and intensity of the program. The design that will initially be discussed is a group skills training model. Groups meet two times weekly for 3 hours with an optional third day for individuals also diagnosed with chemical dependency; this third day is based on a DBT-S curriculum. A clinician does not need to adhere to a specific order for the sessions. The structure of the program provides the clinician with a high degree of flexibility. This allows for individualization and customization of the skills to each individual in the group. Each session is formatted to provide goals for the individual and the group as a whole. There are multiple discussion topics designed to assess the individual's strengths, barriers to effective functioning, and to establish a baseline of understanding and coping. The discussion points can also provide a general orientation and segue to the coping skills. Each session has general coping concepts and specific skill sets for the individual to learn. The individual is taught a set of skills, encouraged to practice in the session, and then move to generalizing the skills to multiple aspects of their lives.

Group/session structure

Section 1: teaching
The group structure of the TAG program is designed to meet twice each week for three hours. Each hour is designed to have a specific focus for the individual and the group as a whole. The first section is the Teaching hour. The section is designed to be 45–50 minutes in length. The teaching section is prioritized as the first section of the day to provide grounding for each individual, establish expectations that all members will be focusing on leaning and applying skills, and to reinforce participation throughout the process. This section introduces the specific goals for the teaching. It starts with an introduction to the topic and why the topic is challenging for individuals. Each individual is engaged in the process to identify if this is a strength area for them or a barrier to more effective functioning. If the individual identifies

the topic as a strength area, they are encouraged to establish a goal of building consistency and a sense of mastery with the skills. If the individual identifies the topic area as a barrier to more effective functioning, they are encouraged to establish a goal of learning the core concepts of the skill sets and create an initial plan and commitment to practice the skills in session. Individuals who are working toward building consistency and mastery may then serve as mentors to those individuals who are newer to the skill sets.

Once the individuals and the group as a whole have set goals, the general topic is discussed from a variety of perspectives. This allows for engagement in the process, general orientation to the topic, and to establish baselines of functioning. Individuals are encouraged to provide examples from their lives as to why and how the topic is relevant. The clinician is encouraged to identify strengths, barriers to effective functioning, needs, and provide a segue to the specific skill sets to be taught. This section is designed to be highly interactive and organic in its process. This is where members discuss the topic's relevancy to their situation and see that they are not isolated in their experience as other members are encouraged to share. This provides a direct grounding experience for many individuals and "normalizes" their reality.

The next section is the skills training component. This is the core of the TAG program. Each session has multiple skill sets to teach. The curriculum is designed to have multiple skill sets that are directly designed to work with the current topic and have generalizability to global coping. This is designed to ground the individual into their current needs, strengths, coping strategies, and global functioning. The next step is to teach specific sets of cognitive and behavioral skills designed to increase the individual's functioning. The skill sets are focused on the current topic and how the individual can learn and apply the skills directly in the session. Each individual incorporates a set of skills into their identified goal work and commits to a plan to generalize the skills into their daily functioning. This plan is then reviewed in the third section where it is problem-solved to address the individual's strengths and barriers.

Section 2: application

The application section is designed to focus on pattern recognition and awareness (based on the principles of self-monitoring and adherence to treatment). The section is designed to be 45–50 minutes in length. A tracking card or diary card is the primary tool used in this section. Each individual completes their tracking card before the session. They review their card with the clinician and the entire group. The card includes areas of functioning, needs, strengths, skills that were used/attempted, and how effective their application of skills have been since the last session. Peers provide feedback in the form of support, challenges, and suggestions to increase effective application and generalizability of the skill sets. Treatment goals and objectives are also reviewed daily in this section.

Section 3: problem-solving

The problem-solving section is designed to assist the individual in applying their strengths to overcome barriers to effective coping. The section is designed to be

45–50 minutes in length. Each individual is expected to identify one of their goal areas that they want to focus on. They take problem-solving time to discuss their strengths, difficulties, their skill implementation plan, commitment to skill use, and receive feedback from the clinician and peers on their action plan. The goal of this section is to have the individual commit to applying their skills outside of the therapeutic setting, create a clear action plan designed to increase the efficacy of their coping strategies incorporating new skills that have been taught in the program, and have a review/completion time established before the next session. The completed action plan is then reviewed in the second section of the next group session. This increases the individual's accountability for follow-through and establishes continuity between sessions.

Curriculum overview

The curriculum is designed to be topic driven (arranged by topic) in an open group format. Therapy is multimodal incorporating group and individual therapy. The program is organized through the Biopsychosocial Model. There are 7 sessions designed to target coping with the biological aspects of mental health and chronic pain; 14 sessions designed to target coping with the psychological aspects of mental health and chronic pain; and 7 sessions designed to target coping with the social aspects of mental health and chronic pain. The term "individual" is used in place of "patient" or "client" to challenge stigma and labels – personalizing therapeutic approaches leads to adherence and personal responsibility.

Sources and recommended readings

It is recommended that the clinician review the original publications and material in the reference section of this manual for further conceptual depth and understanding. I strongly suggest reviewing the works of Steven Hayes on Acceptance and Committment Therapy, William Miller and Stephen Rollnick on Motivational Interviewing, and Marsha Linehan on Dialectical Behavior Therapy.

Biologically based sessions
There are 7 sessions that comprise the focus of skills training designed to target issues related to the biological nature of the individual's mental illness and chronic pain. This section includes:

1. Goal Setting and Motivation
2. Functioning and Loss
3. Sleep
4. Emergence and Patterns
5. Adherence to Treatment Protocols
6. Complexity
7. Working with Your Team

Psychologically based sessions
There are 14 sessions that comprise the focus of skills training designed to target issues related to the psychological nature of the individual's mental illness and chronic pain. This section includes:

1.   Orientation to Change
2.   Readiness to Change
3.   Depression
4.   Anxiety
5.   First Step toward Change
6.   Anger Management
7.   Attending to Distress
8.   Meaning and Pain
9.   Stress Management
10. Defense Mechanisms and Coping Styles
11. Stigma
12. Chemical Abuse
13. Lifespan Issues
14. Managing Flare-ups

Socially based sessions
There are 7 sessions that comprise the focus of skills training designed to target issues related to the social nature of the individual's mental illness and chronic pain. This section includes:

1.   Managing Conflict
2.   The 3 Is
3.   Problem-Solving
4.   Nurturing Support Systems
5.   Social Roles in Relationships
6.   Intimacy
7.   Styles of Interacting

The goals of the program are to reduce hospitalizations, emergency room visits, decrease unnecessary doctor visits, improve individual functioning, improve quality of life, restore hope and activity, decrease demoralization, and reduce overall cost of care for the treatment of the targeted populations.

Suggested program/treatment outcome measures

Treatment Outcome Package (TOP)
The TOP is an outcome measure used to track changes in psychological symptoms and functional domains over the course of treatment. It was developed by Kraus, Seligman, and Jordan (2005) as a comprehensive outcome measurement tool for use in naturalistic settings that could gather information about the full spectrum of presenting problems and psychopathology. Additionally, the TOP collects data about

extraneous variables (e.g., changes in medications, medical illnesses, major life events, etc.) that serve as risk factors with the potential to significantly influence the course of treatment with behavioral health clients (Kraus and colleagues have named these variables *case-mix* variables). The TOP is designed to maximize the chances of measuring meaningful changes in psychological symptoms, functional domains, and case-mix variables over the course of treatment.

The TOP was normed on a large sample of adults with a variety of disorders seeking treatment in a variety of behavioral health services. The TOP generates reports using 12 clinically relevant scales that assist clinicians with (a) diagnosis, (b) treatment planning, (c) outcome assessment, and (d) improving the therapeutic relationship. The 12 clinical scales on the TOP are as follows: Depression, Quality of Life, Psychosis, Panic, Violence, Work Functioning, Mania, Sleep, Substance Abuse, Social Conflict, Sexual Functioning, and Suicidality.

SF-36

The SF-36 is a short form survey that was designed to evaluate health status as part of the Medical Outcomes Study. Initially formed and validated in 1988, it has since been cited in several thousand publications, and has been revised once, in 1996. It provides scores on a scale from 0 to 100 in 8 different domains. These domains are physical functioning, role-physical, bodily pain, general health, vitality, social functioning, role-emotional, and mental health. The reliability of these eight scales and subsequent summary measures have been evaluated in past studies using internal consistency along with test-retest methodology, with a minimum of .70 in the reliability coefficient being found in all but a few studies, and with .80 or higher being standard. The validity of this assessment is supported with various studies indicating that the measure has content, concurrent, criterion, construct, and predictive validity. The SF-36 v1.0 is available for free from the RAND Corporation, and the SF-36 v2.0 is currently controlled and licensed by Quality Metric.

BAP-2

The Behavioral Assessment of Pain Questionnaire (BAP-2) is a self-administered, multidimensional assessment tool for understanding factors that may be working to exacerbate and/or maintain sub-acute and chronic non-malignant pain. The BAP-2 was developed with a normative chronic pain sample of over 1,000 individuals suffering from sub-acute and chronic pain. As a pain assessment instrument, BAP-2 has been shown to have good reliability and validity data (Lewandowski, 2006).

The BAP-2 was developed using a biopsychosocial approach and examines various pain characteristics (e.g., pain intensity, pain behavior, and pain descriptions), past and current levels of physical activity, activity avoidance levels, fears of pain and reinjury, mood, attitudes and beliefs about pain, and behavioral responses to pain. There are over 32 scales that measure such variables as the impact that significant others, such as physicians and family members, may have on the individual's current pain behavior and make appropriate recommendations for successful treatment.

The BAP-2 generates a Clinical Profile report that helps the treating clinician develop a unique treatment plan tailored for that individual. An overall estimate of dysfunction and impairment is estimated for each individual compared to the normative sample.

Quality of Life Questionnaire

The Quality of Life Questionnaire is an assessment tool designed by David Evans, Ph.D. and Wendy Cope, M.A. in 1985 (later published for public use in 1989). Its purpose is to measure "the relationship between a client's quality of life and other behaviors or afflictions, such as physical health, psychological health, and alcohol or other substance use." It contains a total of 192 true/false items, is self-administered, and reportedly takes about half an hour to complete. It can be scored by the administrator and results are provided through five domains (with a total of 15 sub-domains). The major domains are General Well Being, Interpersonal Relationship, Organizational Activity, Occupational Activity, and Leisure/Recreational Activity. It has been used or referenced in approximately 600 studies and has been the subject of several psychometric evaluations to support its validity and reliability. It is available for purchase from Multi-Health Systems and has manual and web-based scoring options.

The Outcome and Session Rating Scales (ORS and SRS)

The ORS and SRS are brief measures for tracking client functioning and the quality of the therapeutic alliance. Each instrument takes less than a minute for consumers to complete and for clinicians to score and interpret. Both scales were developed in clinical settings where longer, research-oriented measures had been in use and deemed impractical for routine use. Versions of the ORS and SRS are available for adults, children, adolescents, and groups in 18 different languages, including French. Individual clinicians may download the scales free-of-charge after registering online at: http://www.scottdmiller.com/?q=node/6. A significant and growing body of research shows the scales to be valid, reliable, and feasible for assessing progress and the alliance across a wide range of consumers and presenting concerns.

Chapter 3

Clinical Manual for
TAG Program

Biological Curriculum

Session focus: Goal setting and motivation

TAG
Teach – Apply – Generalize

- The goal of this session is to
  - Create one goal on each of the three areas: Biological/Psychological/Social
  - Provide feedback from assessment tools/measures and incorporate into the feedback and treatment planning process
  - Personalize client tracking tool for in-session use
  - Learn coping skills to improve the individual's functioning in the areas of goal setting and motivation to cope in a more effective manner
- What to discuss:
  - Setting realistic goals
  - Balancing wants with needs
  - Maintaining commitment to change
  - Introduce relevant forms
- Skills to teach
  - Observe, Describe, Participate
  - Non-judgmental Stance, One-Mindfully, Effectively
  - Radical Acceptance, Practical Acceptance, Practical Change, Radical Change
- Generalize
  - Create an action plan to complete **Goal Setting**
  - Problem-solve barriers
  - Commit to their plan
  - Review in next session
- Review goal sheet

CBT for Chronic Pain and Psychological Well-Being: A Skills Training Manual Integrating DBT, ACT, Behavioral Activation and Motivational Interviewing, First Edition. Mark Carlson.
© 2014 John Wiley & Sons, Ltd. Published 2014 by John Wiley & Sons, Ltd.

Biological Curriculum

Goal setting and motivation

Introduction of the topic

Many individuals want to make changes in their lives. Change is a natural state which allows individuals to be able to adapt, cope, and find enjoyment in life. Individuals are seldom taught how to be advocates for their own change. They may see something that they want and try to get it. When barriers and difficulties arise, individuals often try to continue on their current path until they get what they want, or quit trying because they lose hope. There are fundamental aspects to goal setting that are not formally taught. Education programs do not typically teach steps to goal setting. Life experiences tend to be the primary teacher. Individuals learn in a few basic ways and they can become quite rigid when they are forced to change. It may be easier to do nothing and just accept what is happening. They may feel that what is happening is unjust and respond by fighting against everything. All individuals feel like giving up or fighting everything at times, but extreme reactions tend to be very ineffective. They need to find balance, flexibility, and perseverance to be effective in a consistent manner. Most individuals struggle in three main areas: setting realistic goals, balancing wants with needs, and maintaining their commitment to change.

Setting realistic goals

There are a few key points to review about the process of goal setting. Goals need to be based in reality and they need to be attainable. Many individuals want a cure from their pain or illness. This is not realistic for most people. Hoping for a cure can often create barriers to coping and eventually decrease an individual's ability and desire to cope with their current situation. They need to strike a balance between hope for improvement and the work needed to increase functioning. Chronic health and pain issues can often lead to decreased hope and feelings of disempowerment and inability to necessitate change. Consistent work with goals and objectives can provide the core tools to increase hope and lead to more effective functioning. There are three main steps to setting realistic goals: identifying the Vision of Recovery (VOR), setting the goal, and establishing stepwise and sequential steps to reach the goal (objectives).

Balancing wants with needs

Many individuals struggle with prioritizing their work in treatment. It is natural in the course of treatment to want to focus on the most recent crisis, change in health, or change in functioning. This may be perfectly appropriate for many individuals, but may lead to loss of focus for treatment priorities. The clinician and the individual must agree upon the needs of the individual and prioritize treatment targets as a first step. Once that is done, a Skills Implementation Plan (SIP) form can be completed to target crises that may arise, without losing focus on the treatment priorities. This allows for crisis work in addition to maintaining focus on the agreed-upon treatment targets as changes occur.

   Needs in treatment can be defined as something that is necessary for the individual to live a healthy life. Needs are distinguished from wants because with needs a deficiency would cause a clear negative outcome, such as decreased functioning or increased vulnerability to painful emotions. A want is simply something that a person would like to have. Most individuals struggle with the wish or desire to return to a life free from pain and mental health issues. This is not realistic for most people. Many individuals focus on what they have lost and what they can no longer do. This focus on the past can lead to a variety of painful emotional experiences that results in demoralization and loss of hope. As a consequence, focus and follow-through with treatment recommendations are compromised. Setting goals that are based on needs as opposed to wants is a priority. This encourages the individual to focus more on the present and opportunities for change that can happen in the future. A potential therapeutic benefit is an increase in perceived power and control. The process does not necessarily devalue or invalidate the past, but encourages focus on what can be done now for the individual to be an advocate for positive change in their own lives.

Maintaining commitment to change
Maintaining commitment to change is very difficult for most individuals. Goals and objectives need to have meaning in the individual's life. The clinician is encouraged to establish treatment targets that are relevant to the individual and that are co-created. If goals and objectives are not relevant or are forced upon the individual, motivation and commitment can be compromised. Co-creation of goals allows the individual to choose targets for treatment with the support and guidance of the clinician. The process reinforces a healthy connection without reinforcing tacit agreement by the individual. It may also discourage passive compliance, which is a primary barrier for many individuals. It is important to remember that many individuals have had very little choice in their treatment, procedures, and effects that pain and mental health have had in their lives. The therapist should consult with the individual to agree on initial targets for treatment and throughout the review process for progression in therapy.

Flexibility is another key concept to review with individuals. It is important to challenge all-or-nothing thinking and looking at the world through a black-and-white lens. It is valuable to understand that much of life is lived and experienced between extremes. When individuals are forced to change and have very little choice in this, it is natural to want to simplify what is a very complex process. It is a natural protective process to view life through extremes. A problem arises when extreme views no longer serve a primary protective function and become a barrier to change. Extreme views do not lend themselves well to modification and they generalize to most aspects of life very poorly. The process traps many individuals into thinking that they need to protect themselves from further unanticipated change and they become stuck. They are then more vulnerable to rejection, loss of hope, and invalidation. The clinician needs to validate the extremes and ensure that they serve a purpose at times. The focus can then be turned to other potential options and the pros and cons of making choices or not making them. The goal of flexibility is to provide options and choices that are not accessible to the individual when they are stuck in polarizing extremes.

The last concept for review in this section is the importance of recognizing positives in life. Review the phrase "keep your nose to the grindstone," which means to apply yourself conscientiously to your work. Many individuals also value having a strong work ethic. They need to be cautious about focusing too much on change and moving away from emotional and physical pain too quickly. It is important to remind individuals that the change process is like a marathon and not a sprint. There is value in recognizing the existing positives as well as the positives we are all trying to create in our lives. If individuals hyper-focus on pain and change, they run the risk of losing focus and momentum in treatment. It is important to recognize small steps toward a healthier life. Individuals can challenge their perspective by refocusing on what they want to add to their lives instead of what has been lost. Use terms of "increase" and "gain" instead of "decrease" and "lose." These changes can represent a fundamental shift in thought, behavior, and experience.

Teaching skills (T)

The first set of suggested skills to teach is an overview of the Mindfulness skills from Linehan's DBT manual (1993b). These skills can assist in pattern recognition, awareness, and identification of coping strategies that can be improved. These are important concepts to the creation of therapeutic treatment targets and ongoing skills to use to increase effective coping.

Observe – Noticing one's experience
Describe – The process of putting words on one's experience
Participate – Noting what the individual is doing to cope with the current situation and how present they are in the process

When these skills are used in combination or in a linear fashion, they provide a process to recognize patterns of thoughts and behaviors. They can be used to identify how an individual interprets, reacts, and attempts to cope with an event. This promotes increased awareness of how an individual typically responds to such events.

Non-Judgmental Stance – Noticing our experience without placing judgment on the experience itself or the process
One-Mindfully – Focusing our attention on the present situation or task
Effectively – Doing what is required to meet needs in a healthy manner

When these skills are used in combination with the previous skills they can provide awareness of how effective the individual's attempts to cope are, and can essentially provide a baseline of functioning to start the treatment-planning process.

Acceptance versus change
Marsha Linehan (1993a) introduced the concept of dialectics involving the needed balance of acceptance and change to assist individuals in coping more effectively with difficulties in their lives. Acceptance is the process of acknowledging

something without attempting to change it. It is not the process of quitting or giving up, but rather recognizing the reality of a situation. The reality of the individual is often an effective starting point for engagement in the therapeutic process. Many individuals do not want to accept their current situation and want everything to change. This can lead to unrealistic goals and expectations. Conversely, if we accept everything we will do nothing about our current situation and the result often leads to suffering. A new set of skills will be introduced to target this key concept in treatment which includes: practical acceptance, practical change, and radical change. These skills are designed to assist in the process of setting realistic goals and guide the individual through the process of balancing acceptance and promoting healthy change.

The second set of skills to teach targets the needed balance between acceptance and change. The concept of dialectic may be defined as a commitment to the core conditions of acceptance and change. Progress is made through combining elements that are opposite to one another to create a synthesis based in reality. An example is that I may want to be free from pain (a desire for change), but right now I experience pain on a daily basis (acceptance of what is). If an individual is able to synthesize the truth of both extremes they have an increased ability to view their experience in a more realistic manner. The synthesis may involve a combination of focusing on one or more of the skills outlined in this section.

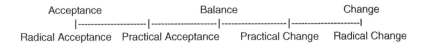

On one end of the dialectic is **Radical Acceptance** (RA). This skill may be defined as accepting reality for what it is. It is letting go of fighting or resisting one's current situation and accepting that attempts to change reality may be futile. This skill is about accepting 100% of the situation while focusing on changing how the individual copes and adapts to the situation itself. That is where power and perceived control are found.

For Example: An individual may need to accept that pain is a part of their everyday life and their current option is to change how they respond to this reality.

A less extreme version of this skill is **Practical Acceptance** (PA). This skill may be defined as accepting reality and understanding that controlling the situation is futile, but realizing that the individual can still influence that situation. They can still change aspects of the situation and how they respond to it. PA is less extreme than RA in the sense that it still implies an acceptance of reality for what it is, but also a recognition that the individual has not exhausted all attempts to influence (change) internal or external factors, which are causing distress. The skill allows for a high degree of acceptance while encouraging appropriate action designed to promote healthy change. The individual may accept 80% (most aspects that are change resistant) of the situation while targeting 20% (some aspects that can be influenced) for change.

For Example: An individual may need to accept that pain is limiting their functioning *and* that they can still modify their activities to change how they respond to this reality.

The next skill on the dialectic is **Practical Change** (PC). This skill may be defined as changing many aspects of a situation and needing to accept some aspects that are change resistant. PC encourages the individual to focus on action and changing the situation itself while they change how they respond. The skill allows for the promotion of a high degree of change while encouraging the acceptance that not all aspects will change. The individual may target change for 80% (most aspects that can be influenced) of the situation while accepting 20% (some aspects that are change resistant).

For Example: An individual may need to change their activity levels due to pain while accepting some limitations that cannot currently be changed.

The last skill on the dialectic is **Radical Change** (RC). This skill may be defined as changing all aspects of a situation because no other alternatives are acceptable. This is an extreme skill designed for application in extreme situations. RC is about changing 100% of the situation while focusing on changing how the individual copes and adapts to the situation itself. That is where power and perceived control are found.

For Example: An individual may need to change their entire approach to treatment if non-compliance or partial-compliance is not effective.

Applying skills and concepts (A)

- Introduce/discuss **Diary or Tracking Cards**
- Introduce/discuss **SIP Form**
- Create safety plans and commitment expectations
- Actively create goals and objectives in session
- Discuss common barriers to this process

Generalizing skills and concepts (G)

- Problem-solve barriers to setting treatment goals and objectives
- Create an action plan for **Goal Setting**

Notes to clinicians and individuals

- Treatment needs to be viewed like a marathon and not a sprint.
- Skills tend to be most effective when used in combinations.
- Three new skills have been introduced to promote healthy coping.
- Treatment goals and objectives are more effective when created WITH individuals, not FOR them.
- Treatment plans are more accepted and promote care when shared and coordinated with the entire treatment team.

Session focus: Functioning and loss

TAG
Teach – Apply – Generalize

- The goal of this session is to
  - Learn coping skills to improve the individual's ability to cope effectively in the areas of daily functioning and loss
- What to discuss:
  - Reinforcement of pain
  - Reinforcement/punishment of healthy activities
  - Loss associated with mental health and pain
- Skills to teach
  - Behavioral mapping
  - Event schedules
  - Modifying activities
  - Building Mastery/Building Positives/Mood Momentum/Instilling Hope
- Generalize
  - Create an action plan to make a positive change through their **SIP Form** or **Diary or Tracking Cards**.
  - Problem-solve barriers
  - Commit to their plan
  - Review in next session
- Review goal sheet

Functioning and loss

Introduction of the topic
Issues with mental health and chronic pain provide many challenges to an individual's functioning. The impact is typically experienced on a daily basis. It is important to explore the question, "What do you get out of having issues with chronic pain?" There may be rewards and reinforcers present that may lead to avoidance patterns. Many individuals may be reinforced for not engaging in healthy behaviors because of pain. This may promote a lack of assertiveness and involve compliance issues. It is important to discuss the key concepts of reinforcement of pain and the reinforcement/punishment of healthy activities.

Reinforcement of pain
Positive reinforcement Many individuals are reinforced for having pain as a part of their daily lives and this may be known or unknown to the individual. Positive reinforcement may be defined as: the adding of a rewarding stimulus to increase a certain behavior or response. An example would be when an individual is experiencing pain and the people in their support system tend to their needs, which feels good to the individual. It is also common that others may do something for the individual that they are able to do for themselves. In this case individuals are reinforced for not caring for themselves and may actually become more passive and dependent on those

around them. Those in their support system then begin to get frustrated and resentful while the individual becomes more passive and dependent.

Negative reinforcement   Many individuals also fall into a trap through avoidance and inactivity. Negative reinforcement may be defined as: the taking away of an aversive stimulus to increase a certain behavior or response. An example of this may be if an individual does not want to mow the lawn, cites that they are experiencing pain which precludes them from engaging in the activity and others complete the task for them. They are reinforced for being inactive by removing the task of mowing the lawn, which they did not want to do. This concept may also promote inactivity, passivity, and dependence.

A negative feedback cycle can develop as pain leads to inactivity and inactivity leads to more pain. Ironically, the new pain an individual experiences can be from inactivity and not necessarily from the original source of pain. This is an important point because many individuals combine all pain into one category: the pain that they have lived with for so long. They may not appreciate that the soreness that comes from increased activity after being sedentary is not their original pain, nor is it coming from their primary source of pain. Many individuals with chronic pain are physically inactive – a tragic irony, because inactivity is a more dangerous enemy than pain. Pain teaches many people to rest and reduce their activities. It seems only natural, but excessive rest may be damaging to the individual. Excessive rest (not using your muscles) may cause not only a loss of muscle strength, but also a loss of flexibility and endurance. The way to combat such deficits is through mild exercise. We have learned from many studies in the field of physiotherapy that when you move less, you begin to lose strength in your muscles. We call this deconditioning. The more you rest, the more your muscles weaken. As time goes on, any activity becomes difficult and causes additional pain. The result of this cycle tends to be increased inactivity, loss of hope, demoralization, depression, increased fears, and anxiety. One of the key concepts for discussion is to ask the individual how they want things to be different through a realistic appraisal of their current abilities.

Reinforcement/punishment of healthy activities

There are many challenges faced by individuals who experience pain. It is important to discuss how individuals are reinforced for healthy activities. This is where individuals build mastery in their lives, experience a sense of accomplishment and competency, and increase hope. This can take the form of compliance to treatment, follow-through with consistent activities of daily living (ADLs), and engaging in activities at a frequency, intensity, and duration that is appropriate to their current abilities.

Some individuals may also be in a system or pattern of functioning where they are actually punished for engaging in healthy activities. Punishment may be defined as: the adding of an aversive stimulus to decrease a certain behavior or response. An example of this concept may be where an individual is told to stop engaging in an activity that they are safe engaging in out of fear of increasing pain levels or increasing their risk of injury. There are many other examples of how individuals are punished for engaging in healthy activities. This is an important discussion point to have individuals generate examples of reinforcement and punishment paradigms. This can serve to ground the individual to their own experience, provide opportunities for validation and acceptance, and provide motivation for appropriate change.

Loss associated with mental health and pain

Many individuals experience multiple losses associated with their mental health and chronic pain. The losses are often experienced on a daily basis. Examples include significant changes in daily functioning; reduced participation in ADLs, focusing on the past and associated negative changes, loss of hope, and demoralization. To cope with the changes many individuals avoid engaging in activities or they overcompensate for the loss. Either response tends to be extreme and does not match the realistic demands of daily living. It is important to discuss that changes in mental health can be addressed through skills training and practice. These skills and concepts are covered in the psychological section of the manual.

Changes in physical functioning can be viewed through the lens of the difference between three forms of pain. Pain that lasts a long time is called chronic and extends beyond the expected period of healing. Pain that resolves quickly when the noxious stimulus is removed or the underlying damage or pathology has healed is called acute. Breakthrough pain is pain that comes on suddenly for short periods and is not alleviated by the individual's normal pain management. It is important to note that individuals cope differently with each form of pain. One of the primary issues to discuss is focusing too much on past functioning rather than on the need to modify current activities. When the individual is ready to focus on their current reality, they are more prepared to identify the role of hope in their lives and may be empowered to accentuate and build positive experiences to gain momentum for healthy change.

Teaching skills (T)

The first sets of suggested skills to teach are designed to target behaviors and activities. The goal is to move toward higher functioning through pattern recognition, engagement in activities, and modification of activities when needed. This session is designed to establish baselines of behaviors, identify coping strategies, and introduce/review tracking forms that will be used throughout the manual.

Behavioral mapping

It is important for the individual to recognize that certain activities lead to either an increase or a decrease in pain. The Pain Scale (see Chapter 4) will be used to establish the individual's daily routine and the role of pain in their lives. The individual is to track their activities throughout the day, note down how they attempted to cope, their levels of pain pre/post intervention, and the location or source of their pain. This form is to be completed daily and reviewed in the second section of the program day.

Event scheduling

It is important to plan and prepare for events that may present barriers to effective functioning. The Skills Implementation Plan (SIP) form is designed to prepare the individual for anticipated activities. The form can be used to identify stressful events and create a concrete skills-based plan to promote effective coping. The individual is to complete the plan early in treatment and modify the plan as they learn and apply coping skills throughout the course of the program. It is common to have individuals identify attempts to cope with stressful situations through a wide variety of strategies. The variations in coping may be categorized into three main areas: fight, flight, and freeze. These are covered in the next section.

Modifying activities

Many individuals struggle with modifying activities. A key point of discussion is to review frequency (F) of the activity, intensity (I) of engagement, and duration (D) of involvement. Introduce the concept of altering aspects of FID through attempts at self-regulation and pacing strategies.

"Fight" is a common coping response that may be defined as: continuing to participate in an activity until its completion regardless of the pain that is experienced or produced. Many individuals tend to cope with events by "powering-through." They tend to disregard their pain triggers and continue with the activity.

"Flight" is a common coping response that may be defined as: disengaging from an activity that begins to trigger a pain response. This may be very healthy at times, but may also lead to stopping an activity out of fear that a pain response may happen. This concept also includes disengaging from an activity in the anticipation that pain may be triggered.

"Freeze" is a common coping response that may be defined as: avoiding any activity that may lead to a pain response. Many individuals choose to avoid activities that have no history of causing pain out of fear that pain may occur, so it is safer to avoid the entire situation.

It is important to introduce a "Behavior Chain" to assist the individual in identifying their responses to activities that may or may not affect their pain levels. This allows for review of the antecedents, the response of the individual, and the generation of behavioral alternatives that target increases in adaptive functioning.

BM, BPE, MM, and instilling hope

The second set of suggested skills to teach targets replacement strategies for ineffective attempts to cope. The goal is to engage the individual in behaviors that lead to an instillation of hope and guard against demoralization.

Building Mastery (BM) – Engaging in activities that have a high probability of success. This leads the individual to experience a sense of competency and perceived control.

Building Positive Experiences (BPE) – Engaging in activities that improve quality of life through the individual experiencing a heightened sense of positive emotions. The more time an individual spends engaging in positive activities, the less time they spend focusing on negative situations.

Mood Momentum (MM) – Noticing and engaging in positive experiences and selecting skills to stay engaged in the activity. It is common for many individuals to disengage in positive activities through the anticipation that "all good things must end." This skill is designed to foster motivation for positive and healthy change.

Applying skills and concepts (A)

- Introduce/discuss a **Diary Card**
- Introduce/discuss **SIP Form**
- Introduce/discuss the **Pain Tracking Card**
- Have each individual generate applications of BM, BPE, and MM in their lives
- Discuss common barriers to this process

Generalizing skills and concepts (G)

- Introduce and assign homework on the tracking tools to be completed and reviewed in the next session
- Problem-solve barriers to completing the tools introduced in this session

Notes to clinicians and individuals

- Behaviors are present because they meet needs. Modification is needed when behaviors are extreme responses to situations that do not generalize effectively.
- It is important to validate and learn from the past while focusing attention on how the individual can cope more effectively in the present moment.
- Contingency management is an important concept to review. The goal is to activate behaviors that have a high probability for success.
- The more an individual is able to focus on the positives in their lives, the less time they have to dwell on negatives.

Biological Curriculum

Session focus: Sleep

TAG
Teach – Apply – Generalize

- The goal of this session is to
  - Learn coping skills to improve the individual's functioning in the areas of building and maintaining healthy sleep patterns
- What to discuss:
  - How sleep patterns affect functioning
  - What are habits and routines?
- Skills to teach
  - Building a routine
  - Maintaining a routine
  - Returning to sleep strategies
- Generalize
  - Create an action plan for **Sleep Hygiene**
  - Problem-solve barriers to creating/maintaining a healthy sleep hygiene
  - Commit to their plan
  - Review in next session
- Review goal sheet

Sleep

Introduction of the topic

It is important to note that this session is designed to create a pattern of functioning. This will take time to establish and can be difficult to maintain. Many individuals struggle with sleep and self-cares. Disruptions in sleep can be caused by a variety of issues from activity levels to poor sleep hygiene. When an individual has difficulty with sleep they may experience fluctuations in mood, decreased energy levels, and decreased participation in self-cares which creates a very destructive cycle. This cycle tends to have a global impact on functioning and may be difficult for the individual to recognize. Management of sleep disturbances that are secondary to mental, medical, or substance abuse disorders should focus on hygiene and the underlying conditions (which are addressed in later sessions). Common treatments include a combination of psychotherapy and medication management.

Teaching skills (T)

Healthy sleep hygiene has many elements common to all individuals, but what works for one person may not work as well for another. One of the keys to success is for the individual to experiment and find which behaviors work best for them. The skills taught in this section are separated into three categories: building a routine, maintaining a routine, and returning the sleep strategies.

Building a routine

There are several elements to building a healthy sleep routine. The individual is encouraged to practice these elements for at least one month in a consistent manner.

1. *Go to bed when you are sleepy*
   Do not force your sleep. It may be helpful to set a consistent time to start your bedtime ritual that assists in preparing you for sleep.
2. *If you do not fall asleep after 20 minutes, you need to get out of bed*
   Find a distraction that does not involve strenuous activity and is short in duration. When you become sleepy, go back to bed. This may require a commitment to this process repeatedly until positive gains are achieved.
3. *Get out of bed at the same time every morning*
   You really want to minimize exceptions to this concept. Consistency is a stepping stone to healthy habits. The more we make exceptions, the harder and longer we have to work.
4. *Establish a bedtime ritual that helps you prepare for sleep*
   Engage in activities that calm the mind and body. Warm baths, scents, meditation, stretching, and reading are all effective examples. Notice that watching television is not on this list!
5. *Keep your bedroom cool, quiet, and dark*
   This promotes the 3 Cs of sleep – cool, calm, and centered.
6. *Keep to your schedule*
   Creating healthy habits takes time and consistency. Over time, you will typically experience deeper, restorative sleep.
7. *Avoid naps if at all possible*
   If you must nap keep it to 10–15 minutes in length

Maintaining a routine

1. *Bed is for sleep so minimize other activities done in your bed*
   Your bed is for sleep, not talking on the phone, watching TV, eating, or working on the computer.
2. *Minimize or stop caffeine intake after mid-afternoon*
   This will assist in keeping you calm and relaxed.
3. *Avoid any alcohol consumption within 6 hours of bedtime*
   Alcohol and deep, restorative sleep do not mix well
4. *Avoid big meals or being too hungry before bedtime*
   It is important to have balance with hunger around bedtime. If you need to eat, moderation is a key.
5. *Avoid exercising 6 hours before bedtime*
   Daily exercise is very important and needs to be done earlier in the day.
6. *Have a plan to cope with worry thoughts*
   Engage in deep breathing, visualization, or progressive muscle relaxation when agitated. Keep a notepad next to your bed to write your worry thoughts down and address them in the morning (practice letting go).
7. *List strategies to get back to sleep*

Focus on relaxing your body and calming your mind. Engage in a quiet, non-stimulating activity.

8. *Consult your doctor*

    This is important to do before starting an exercise program and to assess if your sleep problems require primary medical interventions.

Returning to sleep strategies
- Go to bed only when you are ready to fall asleep. This will increase the probability that you will fall asleep quickly.
- Distinguish between fatigue and sleepiness. Fatigue is a state of low energy, physical or mental. Sleepiness is a state of having to struggle to stay awake. People with insomnia often feel tired but "wired" (i.e., not sleepy) at bedtime.
- If unable to fall asleep, get out of bed and return to bed only when sleepy again.
- Avoid clock watching.
- Address your problems during the day to avoid worrying at night. If you are continually worrying, write the worry down in a journal that is kept next to the bed. Make a commitment to address the worry in the morning.
- Create a list of relaxing activities that can be done at night. If you cannot sleep, engage in an activity and return to bed when feeling sleepy.
- Nighttime activities need to be relaxing and require minimal attention and action.

Applying skills and concepts (A)

- Introduce/discuss sleep as a category on the **Diary Card** or **Pain Tracking Card**
- Introduce/discuss sleep as a target area to be covered on the **SIP Form**
- Create a sleep hygiene plan and commitment expectations
- Discuss common barriers to this process

Generalizing skills and concepts (G)

- Problem-solve barriers to creating a plan for **Sleep Hygiene**
- Introduce and assign homework on the individual's sleep hygiene plan

Notes to clinicians and individuals

- The process of creating a sleep hygiene plan takes time and effort.
- Gaining an increase in quality of sleep is the primary goal.
- There are many barriers that need to be addressed for the plans to be effective – encourage patience.
- It is common for the individual to be unaware of their sleep patterns and the negative impact that the lack of restorative sleep has on their functioning – encourage the individual to discuss this concept with their support system and professional team members.
- Most adults need between 7 and 10 hours of sleep each day.

Session focus: Emergence and patterns

TAG
Teach – Apply – Generalize

- The goal of this session is to
  - Gain insight and understanding into patterns and coping strategies targeting the emergence and ongoing issues/symptoms of an individual's distress
  - Learn coping skills to improve the individual's functioning in the areas of pattern recognition and coping with distress
- What to discuss:
  - Emergence of physical pain
  - Emergence of psychological distress
  - Frequency, Intensity, Duration
- Skills to teach
  - **Baseline Assessment Form**
- Generalize
  - Create an action plan for the **SIP Form**
  - Problem-solve barriers
  - Commit to their plan
  - Review in next session
- Review goal sheet

Emergence and patterns

Introduction of the topic

Every individual's pain story is unique, but most share common elements. Our stories typically involve an injury, genetics, environmental factors, or a combination of triggers. It is important to reflect on how the individual initially attempted to cope with their pain. It may not matter to the individual HOW the pain started because this cannot be controlled; it tends to matter THAT the pain started and has not ended.

The individual may be predisposed (genetically) to develop a certain condition or disorder. This may be the case in more progressive diseases or conditions that have pain as a component. Other individuals have environmental factors as the source of their pain. This may be the case in an injury or medical complication. In both cases the individual learns how to cope with their condition over time. We are taught to cope by our own attempts, through modeling behaviors of those around us, through mass media, and by professionals. Seldom have individuals been taught how to cope in a systematic manner.

It is important to discuss that pain is a natural part of life. It serves a function to motivate the individual to withdraw from damaging situations, to protect a damaged body part while it heals, and to avoid similar experiences in the future. We are genetically engineered to withdraw from and to avoid pain. An example would be pulling your hand away from a hot stove without thinking about it first. We learn from our experiences with pain typically in an episodic or chaotic manner. Most people are in pain quite infrequently and do not have a lot of opportunities to practice effective coping techniques. We engage in life and when we experience pain, we focus on it to try to make it go away. When the pain does not disappear we are forced to attend to it daily and not episodically. This is a crucial shift to understand – because the pain is present on a daily basis and we do not have a lot of coping techniques to deal with it. Naturally we try a few random strategies and find something that works for a short period of time. We tend to try that coping technique as a first resort and begin to rely on it being effective. Seldom does one technique work for all kinds and levels of pain. The individual then creates a pattern of responses that work at times and then fail miserably at others. This leads to a reinforcement schedule that is intermittent and very difficult to change. This leads to more pain, loss of hope, demoralization, and further mental health issues. It creates and feeds a vicious cycle that is very difficult to break. This session is designed to identify patterns in experienced pain and to increase the individual's ability to cope more effectively.

Teaching skills (T)

The set of suggested skills to teach in this session is designed to improve the individual's ability to cope with predictability and uncertainty. Pain can create chaos in an individual's life. It can be both predictable and unpredictable in the same moment. Unpredictable triggers for pain can be very dangerous to the individual by encouraging them to avoid and disengage in activities that may be safe and healthy. It is possible to begin to make the unpredictable more predictable through behavioral analysis. If we apply the concepts of frequency (F), intensity (I), and duration (D) we can increase the probability of predicting our pain responses. This can be accomplished in a few steps designed to create an action plan.

Baseline Assessment Form

1. Establish a baseline of current pain through self-assessment.
    This is where the individual rates their pain on a 10-point scale with 10 being extreme pain and 0 being pain-free. The individual then selects a level of pain that is acceptable to them and at a level where they have effective coping strategies.
2. Review similar past activities by examining the frequency of engagement in the activity and how that affected pain levels.
    This is where the individual recalls similar situations and compares their current functioning to previous functioning when engaging in similar activities. The comparison between past and present may provide information on how frequently they engage in activities before their pain levels are pushed to coping threshold.
    If the probability for increased pain is high, the individual may need to decrease the frequency of engagement in the activity.

3. Review similar past activities by examining the intensity of engagement in the activity and how that affected pain levels.

    This is where the individual recalls similar situations and compares their current functioning to previous functioning when engaging in similar activities. The comparison between past and present may provide information on how intensely they engage in activities before their pain levels are pushed to coping threshold.

    If the probability for increased pain is high, the individual may need to modify the intensity of engagement of the activity through pacing or altering the activity itself.

4. Review similar past activities by examining the duration of engagement in the activity and how that affected pain levels.

    This is where the individual recalls similar situations and compares their current functioning to previous functioning when engaging in similar activities. The comparison between past and present may provide information on how long they can engage in activities before their pain levels are pushed to coping threshold.

    If the probability for increased pain is high, the individual may need to decrease the length of engagement in the activity. They may need to break down the task into smaller parts that can be accomplished over time in stages.

5. Analyze the data and attempt to predict the pain response given past experience and current functioning and ability.

    This is where the individual compares the present situation to what they have learned from the past. They create a probability for increased pain that is low, moderate, or high.

6. Complete a Pros and Cons list for engaging in the activity and for not engaging in the activity.

    This is where the individual decides if the "risk is worth the reward." They also review their current strengths and vulnerabilities.

7. Create/ review their **SIP Form** or coping plan.

    This is where the individual creates or reviews a specific coping plan in relation to the activity.

8. Create the action plan and commit to its implementation.

    This is where the individual acts on their plan with no regret or remorse. They have done their best to analyze the situation and act accordingly.

Applying skills and concepts (A)

- Review the proposed steps of the action plan
- Review the concepts of Pros and Cons
- Introduce/discuss **SIP Form** or create coping plan
- Discuss common barriers to this process

Generalizing skills and concepts (G)

- Problem-solve barriers to the action plan process
- Create an action plan for the **SIP Form**

Biological Curriculum

- Introduce and assign homework on the individual's commitment to the action plan

Notes to clinicians and individuals

- Applying this concept is designed to challenge old behavior patterns and generate new and more effective patterns.
- It is anticipated that themes of fear, anxiety, and avoidance will emerge. It is important to validate an individual's concerns while focusing on what can be done in the present moment.
- Skill sets targeting truly unanticipated pain and flare-ups are covered later in the manual. Focus on the current task and avoid distractions to creating action plans.

Session focus: Adherence to treatment protocols

TAG
Teach – Apply – Generalize

- The goal of this session is to
  - Establish the individual's level of adherence to treatment protocols
  - Assess the individual's strengths and barriers to adherence
  - Learn coping skills to improve the individual's functioning in the area of adherence to treatment protocols
- What to discuss:
  - Adherence to treatment protocols
  - Frustration with medications
  - Frustration with treatment providers
  - Chemical abuse/dependency
  - Self-advocacy
- Skills to teach
  - Dear Man
  - Give
  - Fast
- Generalize
  - Create an action plan for **Self-Advocacy**
  - Problem-solve barriers to adherence to treatment protocols
  - Commit to their plan
  - Review in next session
- Review goal sheet

Adherence to treatment protocols

Introduction of the topic
Adherence to medical treatment protocols may be defined as: the extent to which a person's behavior corresponds with agreed recommendations from a health care provider. Research indicates that up to 60% of individuals who are working on a treatment regimen for chronic conditions demonstrate non-adherence to treatment protocols (Bosworth 2010). The implications of non-adherence include lack of pro-gression in treatment, increased costs of health care, loss of productivity and revenue, the over-utilization of emergency services, more unnecessary doctor visits, and failure to make lasting changes in functioning.

It is unrealistic to expect every individual to follow the agreed-upon treatment protocols 100% of the time. There are many barriers that individuals experience which lead to non-adherence. Many of these barriers can be separated into four categories for easier review and for purposes of discussion.

Frustration with medications
It has been shown that approximately 60% of individuals diagnosed with chronic pain use medications to treat their condition (Bosworth 2010). Many individuals are

frustrated with the effectiveness of medications. There are questions concerning whether the correct medications have been prescribed, whether the right dosages are being administered, and the potential for over-reliance on their use. Frustration levels are also high because of the possible side-effects, dependency issues, and interactions between the medications. Many individuals feel as if they have been prescribed medications that have minimal effects and that they need different interventions to promote lasting change. It has been found that individuals typically underuse, overuse, or abuse their medications when non-adherence is an issue. It is important to raise the issue of adherence to medication protocols to be able to assess for effectiveness and to understand how medication management can assist in stabilizing and potentially improving global functioning.

Frustration with treatment providers

It is a very common experience to be frustrated with the professionals who are involved in the provision of care. Many individuals do not feel as if the providers listen well and understand what they are experiencing. It is common to feel rushed in appointments and to question whether the provider is doing all that they can to provide the best care possible. Many individuals do not feel as if providers believe them when discussing their pain experiences and activity levels. One of the most common experiences is to be frustrated about having little influence in the treatment being provided. Many individuals have unanswered questions and too little information to make effective decisions. Few individuals feel as if they have enough power and control in their treatment. If individuals do not feel as if they are involved in their own care, motivation for adherence decreases significantly.

Chemical abuse/dependency

Chemical abuse or dependency may also present as a primary barrier to adherence to medical protocols. It is common for the individual to miss appointments, have complications in medication management, and engage in protocols intermittently. It is currently believed that chronic pain cannot adequately be treated and may actually get worse if the individual is abusing drugs and/or alcohol. Many treatment providers will provide a referral to formal treatment programs or facilities. Common treatment protocols include intensive medication monitoring, medication contracts, and managing pain with non-opioid and non-pharmacologic interventions. It is common for providers to continue providing services while the individual is in a drug treatment program or facility. This topic will be covered in depth later in the manual.

Self-advocacy

An aspect of self-advocacy is being assertive in a healthy manner. It means taking an active role in treatment protocols. Individuals are encouraged to co-create care and treatment plans. It is important to ask questions and gather as much data as possible to make informed decisions. The individual may also need to assist in the coordination of their own care. Do not be afraid to ask providers if they are sharing information with each other. Make sure that Releases for Personal Health Information (PHI) have been reviewed and endorsed. Know what information can and cannot be shared between providers. The individual is typically in charge of deciding what information can be shared and with whom. Consent to release and share information is required for the team to be able to function to its highest potential.

A second aspect of self-advocacy is being aware of your rights. Every agency is required to have and provide a "Bill of Rights" (BOR) to each individual seeking service. The BOR includes information on the agency's policy and procedures, responsible authorities, data privacy, funding sources, and grievance procedures. To be a strong self-advocate it is important to know your rights. Individuals are often unaware of how their rights may influence their care. It is a common misperception that everybody has equal access to health care. This is not the case! Individuals need to be aware of what health care is available and what procedures or services their insurance covers. Insurance coverage can dictate what services are able to be accessed.

One of the most difficult and challenging areas of health care is being able to engage with multiple providers in an effective manner. Health care professionals are very busy and may not have available time to provide and coordinate all aspects of care. It is imperative that individuals learn self-advocacy skills. One aspect of self-advocacy is being aware of the role that each member has on the treatment team. A typical multidisciplinary team may consist of medical doctors, physician-assistants, nurses, nurse practitioners, physical therapists, occupational therapists, psychiatrists, psychologists, and social workers. Each member of the team has an area of competency and specific set of skills used in the provision of care. It is common for individuals to make a request in a very skillful manner, yet find that the professional does not function in the role to be able to grant the request. They may not have the power, authority, or competency to respond appropriately.

Teaching skills (T)

The sets of suggested skills to teach in this session are designed to increase communication skills and effective participation in medical treatment protocols.

Assertiveness training is a key component to working with medical providers. The first set of skills to teach is an overview of the Interpersonal Effectiveness skills from Linehan's DBT manual (1993b) and modified in Pederson & Pederson's DBT manual (2012). The skill set of **DEAR MAN (DM)** is designed to teach the individual to increase the probability of getting their wants or needs met.

Describe – Use Observe and Describe to summarize the situation and identify the facts that support the request or reason for setting a limit or boundary.
Express – Share your beliefs or opinions when relevant or required.
Assert – Ask clearly for what you want or need.
Reward – Let others know how helping you meet your wants or needs will potentially impact their situation.
Mindful – Stay focused on your request and avoid leaving the topic.
Act confident – Use an assertive tone, have confident body language, make eye contact, and stay calm.
Negotiate – Be willing to compromise to meet your wants or needs.

To apply the skill set of **DM**, the individual must first prioritize their needs. Make sure that the person you are communicating with has the capability of providing for the request. Be aware of asking the right person at the right time. Consider if it is appropriate to ask for something given the status of the current relationship. It is also important to review whether the request meets short-term wants/needs or long-term wants/needs.

This is an important skill set to apply in addressing barriers to adherence. The skill set can assist the individual in advocating to be an active member of their own treatment team. It can also help them to view themselves as a partner with their physicians and service providers. This promotes working together, as a team, toward a common goal. It promotes active participation and a sense of empowerment and ownership. The individual can make a request for clear *written* medication instructions that reduce the risk of underuse, overuse, and abuse. These are all key factors in improving adherence.

The skill set of **GIVE (G)** is designed to teach the individual to build and maintain relationships.

Gentle – Be respectful in your approach and avoid threats, demands, and attacks.
Interested – Listen to the other person and be open to the information they have to provide.
Validate – Acknowledge and attempt to understand the other person's perspective.
Easy Manner – Be political and treat others in a kind and relaxed manner.

This is an important skill set to apply in addressing barriers to adherence. The effectiveness of your medical treatment depends partly on the interpersonal context in which it takes place. It is important to have a healthy, working relationship with the entire treatment team. A wide body of research suggests that a stressful interaction with the individual's physician tends to have a negative impact on overall health and care. The effectiveness of the individual's pain management is influenced by interpersonal styles, the unique interaction the individual has with their physician, and the physician's background, training, and personality.

The skill set of **FAST (F)** is designed to teach the individual how to have self-respect and self-worth.

Fair – Be fair to yourself and others.
Apologies – Do not engage in unnecessary apologetic behavior.
Stick to values – Use your own value system as a guide for your behavior.
Truthful – Be honest and accountable to yourself and others.

This is an important skill set to apply in addressing barriers to adherence. An individual who struggles in this area tends to be passive in their treatment, hesitates to discuss any concerns, does not engage in self-advocacy, does not see themselves as a member of their own treatment team, and lacks motivation for positive change.

Applying skills and concepts (A)

- Discuss **DM**, **G**, and **F** in relation to current adherence levels
- Practice the skills through role-plays

- Problem-solve situations where one skill may be more effective than the others
- Practice discussing the information gathered through the tracking tools to prepare for future medical appointments
- Practice asking for clarifying information
- Practice taking a more active role in your own treatment
- Discuss common barriers to these skills

Generalizing skills and concepts (G)

- Problem-solve barriers to medication compliance
- Problem-solve barriers to taking an active role with the current treatment team
- Problem-solve barriers to medical treatment protocols
- Problem-solve barriers to building and maintaining relationships with health care professionals
- Create an action plan for **Self-Advocacy** (Medical Comprehensiveness)

Notes to clinicians and individuals

- The skills taught in this section take time to become effective.
- Practice is required to build proficiency.
- It may be difficult to prioritize one skill over another. These skills are most effective when applied in combination. The individual may need to start with one skill and then switch to focusing on another to meet the demands of the situation.
- Being skillful means increasing the probability of meeting needs; it does not guarantee a positive outcome.
- The simple act of asking questions and fully understanding what treatment protocols entail is an act of self-advocacy. Taking an active role in treatment leads to empowerment.
- Individuals are experts on and about themselves. Fear, anxiety, and depression may lead them to forget this fact.

Biological Curriculum

Session focus: Complexity

TAG
Teach – Apply – Generalize

- The goal of this session is to
  - ○ Gain insight into and understanding of comorbidity
  - ○ Learn coping skills to improve the individual's functioning in the areas of reporting and symptom expression
- What to discuss:
  - ○ Define complexity
  - ○ *DSM-V*
  - ○ Mental health and chronic pain
- Skills to teach
  - ○ Validation
  - ○ **MY STORY**
- Generalize
  - ○ Create an action plan for **MY STORY**
  - ○ Problem-solve barriers
  - ○ Commit to their plan
  - ○ Review in next session
- Review goal sheet

Individual complexity

Introduction of the topic
Chronic pain, in psychological terms, is a chronic, often overwhelming stressor that has the potential to feed back on itself in a cyclic nature. Chronic stress becomes a part of everyday life when dealing with feelings of loss, grief, fear, and anger. Other psychological concerns with chronic pain and other illness may include vocational problems, cognitive impairments, sexuality response issues, financial concerns, family and social problems, physical discomfort, and excessive worry. Overall, then, comorbidity of psychiatric diagnosis and pain should be viewed as the rule rather than the exception (Kirsh, 2010). According to the field of mental health, comorbidity may be defined as the presence of more than one diagnosis occurring in an individual at the same time. We may also call this comorbidity "complexity" within the individual, in order to challenge potential stigma.

DSM-V
It is important to review how diagnoses are made in the fields of psychology and psychiatry. The Diagnostic and Statistical Manual of Mental Disorders (*DSM*) is currently in its fifth edition. The *DSM* is structured to provide information and clarity on diagnoses. Diagnoses include clinical disorders and other conditions that may be a focus of clinical attention. Examples of common diagnoses include depression, anxiety, bipolar disorder, and schizophrenia among others. There is a list of

symptoms that must be present and specific durations of these symptoms in order for an individual to fit a certain diagnosis. Each diagnosis has a narrative explanation of features, prevalence information, course information, and differential diagnosis.

Other mental health diagnoses address issues such as personality disorders and mental retardation. Examples include dependent personality, borderline personality, and histrionic personality among others. Personality disorders might be characterized as having personality traits and associated behaviors that cause significant distress and loss of functioning when interacting with others. Patterns of behaviors and interaction styles are deeply engrained and are difficult to change.

It is important to consider general medical conditions that might affect the etiology, presence, or worsening of the mental health disorders. It is very common for individuals who experience pain to have a worsening of their negative mood.

Stressors may also have a significant impact on the individual's functioning. It is important to consider daily stressors, life-changing events, and an individual's social support network. Many factors influence an individual's ability to cope with pain and distress. Complexity is a very important factor to address and no individual reacts in a clear, consistent, and predictable manner to changes in functioning.

Mental health and chronic pain

Anxiety, anger, depression, and adjustment disorders are mental health issues commonly related to chronic pain. Many of the symptoms of these disorders are experienced physically and are actually made worse by increases in stress levels. It is important to identify how chronic pain affects mental health and how mental health affects chronic pain. It is important to discuss common reactions to physical and emotional pain. Explore themes of changes in mood, behaviors, and thoughts. Once common reactions are explored, discuss how stress affects the individual's reactions. Identifying how individuals cope with their distress can provide opportunities for validation. It is important for the individual to be able to accept their current reality. The professional can then target aspects of each session from this manual that are relevant to the individual's needs in order to promote effective coping strategies. It all starts with validation (not necessarily acceptance) of their current experience.

Teaching skills (T)

The suggested skill to teach in this session is designed to increase the individual's ability to connect more effectively with their own experience.

Validation – To acknowledge, confirm, authenticate, verify, or prove. This concept may be simple to understand, but is very difficult to apply in a consistent and effective manner to ourselves.

What validation is: Validation is acknowledging your own thoughts, feelings, and experience. Trust yourself and your instincts. There is no room for judgment, interpretation, rationale, or disbelief.

For example: "I am in a lot of pain and my energy levels are really low."

Fact + supporting evidence = confirmation

Fact (I am in a lot of pain) + supporting evidence (my energy levels are really low) = confirmation (distress).

What validation is not: Validation is not agreeing with others or giving in. Do not let others tell you what you think, feel, or are experiencing. This happens when you need to judge, interpret, rationalize, or prove to yourself or someone else that what you are experiencing is real. Stop looking for confirmation through others before seeking it in yourself first.

For example: "I am in a lot of pain, but nobody believes me so maybe I shouldn't feel this way."

Fact + interpretation = invalidation

Fact (I am in a lot of pain) + interpretation (nobody believes me) = invalidation (maybe I shouldn't feel this way)

Applying skills and concepts (A)

- Practice validating your thoughts
- Practice validating your emotions
- Practice validating your pain
- Practice validating your behaviors
- Practice validating your experience
- Problem-solve barriers to this process

Generalizing skills and concepts (G)

- Problem-solve barriers to practicing and applying self-validation
- Assign homework to practice this skill on a daily basis and report on its effectiveness
- Assign the first ½ of **MY STORY**

Notes to clinicians and individuals

- "You are not your diagnoses" is an important topic to discuss.
- It is common to have multiple diagnoses when dealing with chronic health issues.
- Validation takes practice, practice, practice to apply effectively.
- Validation is not accepting the current situation; it is acknowledging that it exists.
  - Accepting situations can lead to non-action and to accepting things that need to be changed.

Session focus: Working with your team

TAG
Teach – Apply – Generalize

- The goal of this session is to
  - ○ Increase self-advocacy in an effective manner
  - ○ Gain information and insight into working with multidisciplinary teams
  - ○ Learn coping skills to improve the individual's functioning in the area of working with professionals
- What to discuss:
  - ○ Working with your team
  - ○ Preparing for appointments
  - ○ Engaging in complaining behaviors
- Skills to teach
  - ○ Preparing for an appointment
  - ○ **KEEP IT REAL**
- Generalize
  - ○ Create an action plan for **KEEP IT REAL**
  - ○ Problem-solve barriers
  - ○ Commit to their plan
  - ○ Review in next session
- Review goal sheet

Working with your team

Introduction of the topic
Regardless of the intentions of physicians, studies have shown that they tend to take those people in acute pain and those with cancer more seriously to those with chronic non-malignant pain. A Michigan study of 368 physicians looked at how patient characteristics influenced physician behaviors (Green *et al.*, 2011) and found that physicians were more likely to provide optimal treatment for men with acute post-operative or cancer pain. Physicians reported lesser goals for relief of chronic pain when compared to acute and cancer pain. This information highlights the importance of working effectively with professionals who are part of your care. It is important to discuss the topics of preparation for appointments and engagement in complaining behaviors. These areas can be barriers to receiving effective care, but can be navigated successfully when done in a thoughtful and planned manner.

Preparation for appointments
There are many barriers individuals experience when preparing for medical appoint-ments. There may be a delay between the time that a need arose and the actual time of the appointment. This delay can lead to forgetting to attend, forgetting why the appointment was scheduled in the first place, and changes in symptoms and needs over time. The day of the appointment may also be chaotic due to transporta-tion, childcare, the weather, and pacing of travel to the appointment. Individuals

also struggle with presenting clear and concise information to professionals. Individuals often use global and generic language to describe what they are experiencing. This can lead the professional to make inferences and assumptions that may or may not be accurate. Another area that individuals struggle with is identifying clear goals and objectives for each appointment. When the structure and process of the appointment are left to the professional, the individual may not get their needs and wants met.

Engaging in complaining behaviors

It can be demoralizing to be in different forms of pain and discomfort on a daily or weekly basis. It is natural to become frustrated with the process itself and the providers you are working with. Many appointments start with the individual discussing their struggles and frustrations with their treatment protocols and providers. It is important to understand the natural reactions of people when they are dealing with someone who is frustrated. It is normal to become defensive, mirror their emotional state, and have a strong desire to distance oneself from the perceived negativity. Compare the situation to someone working in the lost luggage department at an airport terminal. People who have lost their luggage tend to use negative language, make demands, or have requests that cannot be immediately fixed, and this tends to put pressure on the worker to act quickly in a situation that takes time to understand and resolve. There is a lot of pressure to perform, which leads to high burnout rates and job turnover. It is important to remember that professionals have a job to do and individuals can influence how others treat them. Once an individual is identified as being a "complainer," it is a hard label to change.

Teaching skills (T)

The set of suggested skills to teach in this session are designed to increase the individual's ability to work with professional team members in an effective manner.

Preparing for appointments is a very important activity. The individual can structure a set of tasks to complete before the day of the appointment.

1. Prioritize needs and wants – Brainstorm a sheet of needs and wants. Organize them into a list with priorities being at the top.
2. Set clear goals and objectives for the appointment – Know the purpose of the meeting and specifically what you want to accomplish before the meeting ends.
3. Create a list of questions for the professional – Organize your thoughts into a list of questions. Post them in an area that you frequently spend time in so you can add questions to the list as you think of them.
4. Organize the tracking forms and tracking cards – Gather the most recent and relevant information you have. This is one way to avoid seeming forgetful or vague.
5. Plan for childcare if needed – Ask a friend, family member, or the professional's facility to assist. It is important to be able to focus your attention and be mindful during the appointment.

6. Plan or coordinate transportation – Make sure you have a reliable plan and mode of transportation. This is one of the first reasons individuals miss appointments.
7. Plan for an advocate to attend if needed – Bring something to take notes on during the appointment. If this is difficult, ask if a friend or family member can attend to help you.
8. Visualize the appointment – Imagine yourself staying focused, active, and productive in the meeting. This will help increase your chances of getting your needs met.

Structuring the day of the appointment can assist in this process as well.

1. Confirm childcare – Avoid last-minute chaos where possible.
2. Gather materials – Do not leave them at home.
3. Review the goals and objectives for the appointment – Remind yourself of the reasons for the appointment and what you want to accomplish.
4. Engage in a stress-management exercise – Take some time to relax and breathe before the appointment. Deep breathing, progressive muscle relaxation, and imagery can help to calm your nerves.
5. Leave at an appropriate time – Plan to be about 10–15 minutes early to your appointment. Being late can compromise your chances of having a productive appointment.

During the appointment, remember to **KEEP IT REAL**.

1. **K**ey in on the task at hand – You are attending an appointment with a professional. Be respectful and take an active role in your care.
2. **E**stablish the goals for the appointment – State your goals at the start of the appointment. It will be clear that you are taking an active role in your treatment and may help in structuring the appointment.
3. **E**stablish the available time – Ask the professional how long they *realistically* envision the appointment taking and pace yourself accordingly.
4. **P**rovide information – Present your tracking tools and the information you have gathered. This may also include your written list of questions. Be clear and specific.
5. **I** statements – Make consistent "I" statements and take responsibility for your decisions and care.
6. **T**ake notes – Write down the answers to your questions to help you remember them. You can also review them later.
7. **R**equest written materials – Gather as much information as you can. Information helps with making decisions and motivation.
8. **E**ngage in reflective communication – When a question is answered or you need clarity, let the professional know what you heard and check to make sure your interpretation and memory are accurate.
9. **A**sk questions – Be assertive. No question is too silly or stupid to ask. Do not leave the appointment with unanswered questions.
10. **L**eave with a clear care plan – Know what the next steps in your care are and discuss them with the professional before leaving.

The next set of skills is designed to help individuals avoid over-complaining to professionals and are from Pederson's DBT manual (2012). These skills include **Grounding Yourself (GY), Willingness (W),** and **Non-judgmental Stance (NJS).** The combination of these skills may assist the individual in staying focused on their goals, increase their options, and challenge the role of judgment in their current situation.

Grounding Yourself (GY) – Grounding exercises bring you back to the here and now. This skill can be used to remind the individual to focus on their goals, be respectful, and be reasonable. Focus the individual's attention on the current situation and what behaviors are required in the moment.

Willingness (W) – Meeting others and situations where they are at instead of where we wish they were. This skill can be used to challenge all-or-nothing thinking. It encourages the individual to be open to all options that are being discussed.

Non-judgmental Stance (NJS) – Understanding when to use judgments and when to let them go. This skill can be used to challenge viewing things as "right" or "wrong" or "good" or "bad." Judgments lead to rigid thinking and acting on emotions that tend not to fit the facts of the situation. Look for the shades of gray to explore potential options.

Applying skills and concepts (A)

- Introduce/discuss the homework assignment on **Preparing for an Appointment**
- Introduce/discuss the homework assignment on **KEEP IT REAL**
- Role-play attending an appointment
- Problem-solve barriers to this process

Generalizing skills and concepts (G)

- Problem-solve barriers to creating a plan for attending an appointment
- Introduce and assign homework on the individual's appointment plan

Notes to clinicians and individuals

- Remind individuals to help their team to help them.
- Being prepared for an appointment increases the probability of having wants and needs met.
- Remind individuals to be as specific as possible when completing their tracking cards and conveying information to health care professionals.
- Keep a file for treatment protocols and tracking tools to be able to share with the entire treatment team.
- Do not assume that all members of the treatment team have all the information they need to make decisions.

- Treating others respectfully encourages them to treat you in the same manner.
- Remind the client to be cautious of making emotion-based decisions. Such decisions tend to be impulsive and focused on meeting short-term needs at the risk of damaging long-term relationships.
- Do not forget to thank your team for participating in your care.

Biological Curriculum

Psychological Curriculum

Session focus: Orientation to change

TAG
Teach – Apply – Generalize

- The goal of this session is to
  - Gain insight and information about the impact that perceived control has in coping with change
  - Learn coping skills to improve the individual's functioning in the area of coping with change
- What to discuss:
  - The concepts of control and influence
  - Define Locus of Control
  - How perceived control influences functioning and how it affects approaches to treatment
- Skills to teach
  - Observe
  - Describe
  - Participate
  - Effectively
- Generalize
  - Create an action plan for **CONTROL versus INFLUENCE**
  - Problem-solve barriers
  - Commit to their plan
  - Review in next session
- Review goal sheet

Orientation to change

Introduction of the topic
If an individual feels that they have some control in a situation, they are more apt to act and advocate for themselves. If the same individual believes that they have little to no control, they may become quite passive or even resistant. Every person has tendencies in how they respond to situations. It is important to note not whether these tendencies are "right" or "wrong," but whether they are effective for the individual or not. One way of viewing these tendencies is to explore them through the concept of Locus of Control (Rotter, 1954).

Orientations

Internal Locus of Control
An Internal Locus of Control may be defined as the degree to which an individual believes that they can control their own lives. Individuals who have a high internal

locus of control believe that they are free to live their own their lives, find or create choices to advocate for themselves, and take responsibility for their actions. Freedom, choice, and responsibility are key aspects to improved health.

How a person reacts to change is important to the treatment of both physical and mental health. Change may be planful. An individual can set realistic goals and steps to reach those goals. They can identify strengths to assist them in the challenges that change presents. They can anticipate barriers to change and react accordingly. An example of this may be applying for employment. There are certain steps to take to change job status. An individual typically starts this process by researching what jobs are available and if they will qualify for the application process. They may gather documents, complete an application, schedule an interview, and complete the process. This reaction to change is self-driven, planful, and proactive.

External Locus of Control
An External Locus of Control may be defined as the degree to which an individual believes that their decisions and life are controlled by environmental factors that they cannot influence. Individuals who have a high external locus of control believe that they have little freedom in their lives and tend to feel trapped, that others make decisions for them, and that others are responsible for how things affect them.

There are also instances where change is forced upon an individual. This may not allow for planning before the change actually happens. Individuals are forced into a position where others are more powerful than they are in their own lives, where they are presented with others' plans for them, and where they are reacting to a situation instead of shaping it in a proactive manner. An example of this may be an individual who is recovering from an injury-related accident. They immediately become a "patient" or "client" and have a team of professionals who are responsible for providing treatment or services. The professionals have more knowledge and expertise than the individual does. The professionals explain options and suggest plans for interventions and care. The individual is forced to react to the situation.

Control versus influence

It is important to identify how the individual perceives control in their lives and how this perception or belief affects their functioning. Control may be defined as having power over something. A common belief is that if a person views himself or herself as "being in control," they SHOULD be able to exert their power and force change. This can be very positive when the change that a person desires can become reality through their efforts. "I will find a way or make it!" is a great example of how this perception can lead to positive action. A problem arises when the situation or an individual's response is resistant to being controlled. If they attempt to exert their power and do not get the desired result, they become polarized in their interpretation. "I failed." "I needed to work harder or do more." Polarized interpretations lead to all-or-nothing and black-and-white thinking. This reduces freedom of acceptable experience, restricts choices, and makes it difficult for the individual to take responsibility for their actions. This may become clearer through a common example. Many individuals believe that they can "control" their emotions. If emotions could truly be controlled, there would be no use for medication-management or psychotherapy. The individual would simply exert their power and choose not to be depressed or anxious. If this ability were true, depression and anxiety would not be related to chronic pain. The belief that things can be controlled implies that there is a clear and predictable course of action that leads to one acceptable outcome. This belief does not generalize well to the reality that most individuals experience.

Influence may be defined as producing some effect without exerting direct control or power. If the individual focuses their attention on exerting influence, they have more choices and possibilities. This challenges all-or-nothing and black-and-white thinking. This concept can be clarified by continuing the example in the previous paragraph. Replace the belief that emotions can be controlled with the belief that emotions can be influenced. This change implies that there is no ONE clear course of action that leads to ONE acceptable outcome. The individual does not have to be perfect in their approach to the situation and can accept that change is a process that is dynamic and unpredictable at times. This shift in belief allows for flexibility in beliefs, interpretations, choices, actions, and acceptable outcomes. There is now a range of what is allowable or acceptable which makes it easier for the individual to take responsibility for their actions and involvement in the process.

Teaching skills (T)

The set of suggested skills to teach in this session is designed to increase the individual's perceived sense of control.

Observe – Noticing one's experience
Describe – The process of putting words on one's experience

This set of skills will provide a pattern of *interaction* that will assist in identifying the individual's Locus of Control. When these skills are used in combination or in a linear fashion, they provide a process to recognize patterns of thoughts and behaviors. They can be used to identify how an individual interprets, reacts, and attempts to cope with an event. This promotes increased awareness of how an individual typically responds to events.

Participate – Noting what the individual is doing to cope with the current situation and how present they are in the process
Effectively – Needs are being met in a safe and healthy manner. This skill is important to teach and review when identifying whether the individual's current functioning is optimal or acceptable.

This set of skills will provide a pattern of *functioning* that will assist in identifying the individual's potential need for modifying their coping patterns. Is what they are doing (participate) meeting their needs in a safe and healthy manner (effectively)? If the answer is yes – reinforce the pattern of behavior. If the answer is no – problem-solve barriers to effective functioning.

Applying skills and concepts (A)

- Introduce/discuss the homework assignment on **CONTROL versus INFLUENCE**
- Problem-solve barriers to this process

Generalizing skills and concepts (G)

- Assign individuals the task to complete the open sections of the homework
- Assign the individual the task to review their work with their support system and treatment team

Notes to clinicians and individuals

- Changing the individual's Locus of Control is NOT the goal of this session. It is designed to review their functioning and increase their effectiveness in getting their needs met in a safe and healthy manner through skill application.
- Challenge all-or-nothing and black-and-white thinking by identifying when it is a barrier to freedom of experience, or is restricting choices and making it difficult to take responsibility. Then healthy alternatives can be explored.
- Validate that there are times when external factors are more influential and powerful than the individual.
- Perception is reality – keep this in mind when working with individuals who feel stuck in behavior patterns and have difficulty identifying options and potential for change.

Psychological Curriculum

Session focus: Readiness to change

TAG
Teach – Apply – Generalize

- The goal of this session is to
  - Identify where individuals are in the change process while assessing for motivation to progress and make changes in their lives
  - Learn coping skills to improve the individual's functioning in the areas of motivation and change
- What to discuss:
  - Change
  - Distress and overall functioning
  - Stages of change
- Skills to teach
  - Observe, Describe, Participate
- Generalize
  - Create an action plan for reviewing/modifying treatment plans
  - Problem-solve barriers
  - Commit to their plan
  - Review in next session
  - Review **Readiness** to Change handout
- Review goal sheet

Readiness to change

Introduction of the topic
Change is a natural part of life. When individuals are experiencing challenges in their lives due to changes in physical and emotional health, their lives may feel extremely chaotic. In the midst of the chaos, there are patterns of functioning that emerge. It is important to identify these patterns to be able to address specific issues instead of targeting aspects that are vague and difficult to identify. A point of discussion is that we experience change whether we want to or not. How individuals react to change is a key clinical issue to target. We may be in different stages of change with each separate issue or even certain aspects of coping and functioning. The individual's engagement in the treatment process has a direct impact on appropriateness for care, what protocols may be effective, compliance to treatment, and motivation for change. Before this concept is explored in depth, it is important to provide a context for discussion. This can be done by exploring how distress affects overall functioning.

Distress and overall functioning
If an individual is in a state of high distress, they may respond by being reactive, desperate, and impulsive. This leads to a decrease in functioning and effective coping if the distress is experienced over long periods, as in the case of chronic pain and illness. One of the keys to dealing with this concept is to teach the individual skills,

and to hold them accountable to practicing them consistently. Through consistent skill work, it is anticipated that the individual's distress will reduce, functioning will improve, and that they will experience a higher quality of life.

Stages of change
Researchers (Kerns, Rosenberg, Jamison, Caudill, & Haythornthwaite, 1997) have identified stages of change in relation to individuals experiencing chronic pain. There are four stages to review in this session.

1. Precontemplation stage (Not Ready)
   Individuals embrace beliefs that the pain problem is medical, that medical professionals are expected to relieve it, and that learning self-management skills is useless.
2. Contemplation stage (Getting Ready)
   Individuals recognize the potential usefulness of self-management, but are reticent to abandon the search for a medical cure.
3. Action stage (Doing)
   Individuals in an action stage accept the need for a self-management approach, and are encouraged in efforts to acquire new skills to enrich existing ones.
4. Maintenance phase (Relapse Prevention)
   Individuals have a well-established belief in the usefulness of self-management, and intend to continue consolidating and expanding their skills.

Teaching skills (T)

The set of suggested skills to teach in this session is designed to increase the individual's ability to identify their readiness and orientation to change. It is important to integrate the two concepts and apply them to both physical and psychological functioning.

Observe – Noticing one's experience
Describe – The process of putting words on one's experience
Participate – Noting what the individual is doing to cope with the current situation and how present they are in the process

When these skills are used in combination or in a linear fashion, they provide a process to recognize patterns of thoughts and behaviors. They can be used to identify how an individual interprets, reacts, and attempts to cope with an event. This promotes increased awareness of how an individual typically responds to events.

This set of skills can be used to identify where the individual is in the stages of change process. It is important to separate physical and mental health. Individuals can identify their current physical abilities and challenges. They need to review their treatment and care plans. This will provide the context for their current participation in their health-care. The second step is to have the individual repeat this process concerning their mental health. Once this has been completed, they can apply the skill of **Effectively**.

Psychological Curriculum

Effectively – Needs are being met in a safe and healthy manner

This skill is important to teach and review when identifying whether the individual's current functioning is optimal or acceptable. Observe, describe, and participate provides information about patterns and where the individual is in the stages of change process. Effectively provides information about how effective the individual is being. If what they are doing meets their needs in a safe and healthy manner, continue the plan. If what they are currently doing does not meet these criteria, review and potentially modify their plan.

One way of engaging this process is to have the individual complete a self-assessment on their current functioning levels in physical and mental health. Then have them review their assessment with their support system and with professionals who are currently working with them on their care plans. This process is intended to provide points for discussion, challenge viewpoints, increase insight, and coordinate efforts and care. It may also assist the individual in identifying whether their current situation and responses are acceptable and effective for themselves and others, or if modification is needed.

Applying skills and concepts (A)

- Introduce/discuss the homework assignment on identifying stages of change for both physical and mental health functioning
- Have individuals review the model explained in this session and have them explain it to you or to each other to gain a higher degree of understanding of the terms and concepts
- Problem-solve barriers to this process

Generalizing skills and concepts (G)

- Problem-solve barriers to continuing or modifying their coping and care plans
- Review the level of engagement in their treatment with their support system and professionals involved in their care

Notes to clinicians and individuals

- It is important for individuals to understand that distress reduces their ability to cope and function effectively.
- Each individual is willing to change something in their lives. Start with what they are willing to do. Then you can move toward clinical goals and objectives by building on their strengths rather than challenging them directly or setting goals that they do not believe in.
- Distress and functioning have an inverse relationship.
- Each individual may be at a different stage of change with each issue, or aspects of an issue.
- This work leads to increased insight, motivation, and hope.
- It is important to integrate the process of change with the stages of change. This integration suggests that in the early stages, people apply cognitive, affective, and

evaluative processes to process through the stages. In later stages, people rely more on commitments, conditioning, contingencies, environmental controls, and social support for progressing toward termination (Prochaska &Velicer 1997).

- If an individual is not progressing as anticipated, please reference the session labeled: *First step toward change*
- It is important to read Stuart's (2008) work regarding IPT (Interpersonal Therapy). Many of the concepts addressing change are based on IPT principles. Glenn & Burns (2003) have provided source material for self-management concepts.

Session focus: Depression

TAG
Teach – Apply – Generalize

- The goal of this session is to
  - Identify signs and symptoms of depression
  - Learn coping skills to improve the individual's functioning in the area of depression
- What to discuss:
  - Rates of depression in the chronic pain population
  - Define depressive disorders and common signs and symptoms
- Skills to teach
  - Safety
  - Build Positive Experiences
  - Just Noticeable Change
- Generalize
  - Create an action plan for **Scheduling Positive Events**
  - Problem-solve barriers
  - Commit to their plan
  - Review in next session
- Review goal sheet

Depression

Introduction of the topic
Symptoms of depression are a common experience for individuals who experience chronic pain. Studies indicate that 60%–70% of individuals diagnosed with chronic pain will also meet the *DSM-V* diagnostic criteria for depression. Research has shown that depression is influenced by both biological and environmental factors. Studies show that first-degree relatives of people with depression have a higher incidence of the illness, whether they are raised with this relative or not, supporting the influence of biological factors. Situational factors can exacerbate a depressive disorder in significant ways. Examples of these factors would include lack of a support system, stress, illness in self or loved one, legal difficulties, financial struggles, and job problems. These factors can be cyclical in that they can worsen the symptoms and act as symptoms themselves.

Common symptoms
Symptoms of depression include:

- depressed mood (such as feelings of sadness or emptiness)
- reduced interest in activities that used to be enjoyed
- sleep disturbances (either not being able to sleep well or sleeping too much)
- loss of energy or a significant reduction in energy level

- difficulty concentrating, holding a conversation, paying attention, or making decisions that used to be made fairly easily
- suicidal thoughts or intentions

Treatment

Treatment can either combine pharmacotherapy and psychotherapy or utilize one or the other individually. Medications used to treat this disorder include Prozac, Paxil, Wellbutrin, and Zoloft. Psychotherapy is useful in helping the individual understand the factors involved in either creating or exacerbating the depressive symptomotology. Personal factors may include a history of abuse (physical, emotional, and/or sexual), ineffective coping skills, and physical health. Environmental factors involved in this disorder include, among others, a poor social support system and difficulties related to finances or employment.

Prognosis

Major depressive disorder has a better prognosis than other mood disorders in that medication and therapy have been very successful in alleviating symptomotology. However, many people diagnosed with this disorder find that it can be episodic, in that periodic stressors can bring back symptoms.

Depressive disorders

Major depressive disorder   According to the *DSM-V*, a person who suffers from major depressive disorder must have depression symptoms such as having a depressed mood or a loss of interest or pleasure in daily activities consistently for at least a two-week period. This mood must represent a change from the person's normal mood; social, occupational, educational, or other important functioning must also be negatively impaired by the change in mood. A depressed mood caused by substances (such as drugs, alcohol, medications) or that is part of a general medical condition is not considered to be major depressive disorder. Major depressive disorder cannot be diagnosed if a person has a history of manic, hypomanic, or mixed episodes (e.g., a bipolar disorder) or if the depressed mood is better accounted for by schizoaffective disorder and is not superimposed on schizophrenia, schizophreniform disorder, delusional disorder, or psychotic disorder. Further, the symptoms are not better accounted for by bereavement (i.e., after the loss of a loved one) and the symptoms persist for longer than 2 months or are characterized by marked functional impairment, morbid preoccupation with worthlessness, suicidal ideation, psychotic symptoms, or psychomotor retardation.

This disorder is characterized by the presence of the majority of these symptoms:

- Depressed mood most of the day, nearly every day, as indicated by either subjective report (e.g., feels sad or empty) or observation made by others (e.g., appears tearful). (In children and adolescents, this may be characterized as an irritable mood.)
- Markedly diminished interest or pleasure in all, or almost all, activities most of the day, nearly every day

- Significant weight loss when not dieting or weight gain (e.g., a change of more than 5 pounds of body weight in a month), or decrease or increase in appetite nearly every day.
- Insomnia or hypersomnia nearly every day
- Psychomotor agitation or retardation nearly every day
- Fatigue or loss of energy nearly every day
- Feelings of worthlessness or excessive or inappropriate guilt nearly every day
- Diminished ability to think or concentrate, or indecisiveness, nearly every day
- Recurrent thoughts of death (not just fear of dying), recurrent suicidal ideation without a specific plan, or a suicide attempt or specific plan for committing suicide.

Persistent depressive disorder (dysthymia)　According to the *DSM-V*, dysthymia is characterized by an overwhelming yet chronic state of depression, exhibited by a depressed mood for most of the days, for more days than not, for at least two years. (In children and adolescents, mood can be irritable and duration must be at least one year.) The person who suffers from this disorder must not have gone for more than 2 months without experiencing two or more of the following symptoms:

- poor appetite or overeating
- insomnia or hypersomnia
- low energy or fatigue
- low self-esteem
- poor concentration or difficulty making decisions
- feelings of hopelessness

In addition, no Major Depressive Episode has been present during the first two years (or one year in children and adolescents) and there has never been a Manic Episode, a Mixed Episode, or a Hypomanic Episode, and criteria have never been met for Cyclothymic Disorder. Further, the symptoms cannot be due to the direct physiological effects of the use or abuse of a substance such as alcohol, drugs or medication, or a general medical condition. The symptoms must also cause significant distress or impairment in social, occupational, educational, or other important areas of functioning.

Adjustment disorder　An adjustment disorder is characterized by the development of emotional or behavioral symptoms in response to an identifiable stressor (or stressors) occurring within 3 months of the onset of the stressor. A stressor is anything that causes a great deal of stress in the individual's life. It could be a positive event, like a wedding or purchasing a new home, or a negative event, like the death of a family member, the breakup of an important relationship, or loss of a job.

These symptoms or behaviors are clinically significant, as evidenced by either of the following:

- Marked distress that is in excess of what would be expected from exposure to the stressor
- Significant impairment in social, occupational, or educational functioning

The stress-related disturbance does not meet the criteria for another specific mental disorder. Once the stressor (or its consequences) has ended, the symptoms do not persist for more than an additional 6 months. By definition, if feelings related to the event last longer than 6 months, it will no longer qualify for an adjustment disorder diagnosis.

An adjustment disorder can occur at any time during an individual's life and there is no difference in the frequency of this disorder between males and females. An adjustment disorder is diagnosed by a mental health professional through a clinical interview.

Adjustment disorders are often diagnosed when it is not clear whether the individual meets the criteria for a more severe disorder, or when the actual diagnosis is uncertain. This diagnosis often gives the clinician time to further evaluate the individual during additional therapy sessions.

Teaching skills (T)

The set of suggested skills to teach in this session is designed to increase the individual's ability to cope more effectively with symptoms of depression. The goal is to have the individual engage in activities that create positive reactions in mood and provide distractions from distress.

Safety
The first priority is to assess for safety in all individuals. If the individual is experiencing suicidal ideation this must be addressed before any other issues. If the individual cannot guarantee his or her own safety, a psychiatric hospitalization needs to be considered. If the individual is willing to work on keeping himself or herself safe, a contract can be initiated (see Appendix – Safety Contract). This is also a primary clinical target for the SIP (Skills Implementation Plan) form. A clear commitment to safety is a primary requirement for continued therapy.

Building Positive Experience (BPE) – Creating or engaging in activities that lead to positive moods. This skill is designed to activate behaviors that serve two distinct purposes. It can activate behaviors that lead to positive emotions, which is the primary goal. This promotes healthy activity and leads to more positive moods. This skill can also be used to modify activities that have been avoided or stopped due to the impact of physical pain. The key is to have the individual modify their engagement in the activity instead of not participating in it at all. Modifying activities can also challenge the individual's patterns of all-or-nothing and black-and-white thinking.

Just Noticeable Change (JNC) – Engaging in a behavior that leads to a change in focus or direction. This is a "baby-steps" skill. JNC allows for taking a first step toward change. It is a short-term skill designed to change the individual's "threshold" of experience. This helps the individual to identify that small steps can have a big impact concerning the process of change. The goal is to have the individual do something different to change their current mood. This does not need to be a positive event, but can be neutral. Many individuals actually practice their current mood (listening to sad music which makes depressive symptoms worse) whether they are aware of it or not. JNC encourages the individual to break their thought or behavior cycle by doing something different. Many depressed individuals avoid positive activities because they believe such activities will not affect their mood, are too challenging, or because they believe they are not worth the positive emotion.

Applying skills and concepts (A)

- Introduce/discuss the homework assignment on **Scheduling Positive Events**
- Problem-solve barriers to this process

Generalizing skills and concepts (G)

- Problem-solve barriers to creating a plan for completing **Scheduling Positive Events**
- Have individuals share their plan with their support system for backup and commitment

Notes to clinicians and individuals

- JNC is a new skill to introduce which activates different behaviors that are designed to interrupt negative cycles.
- Many symptoms of depression may be reactions to physical health issues.
- Safety is the first priority in treatment.
- Change can be difficult so engage the individual's support system for assistance.
- It is important to review the skills from the "anxiety" session since many of the skills will work with different forms of emotional distress.
- Identify, validate, and reinforce small changes. They are building blocks for success.
- It is important to review the diagnostic criteria for mental health disorders with individuals. Many have been diagnosed and have not had an explanation as to why.

Session focus: Anxiety

TAG
Teach – Apply – Generalize

- The goal of this session is to
  - Identify signs and symptoms of anxiety
  - Learn coping skills to improve the individual's functioning in the area of anxiety
- What to discuss:
  - Rates of anxiety in the chronic pain population
  - Defining anxiety disorders and common signs and symptoms
- Skills to teach
  - Distracting the Mind, Imagery, Soothing through the Senses
  - PLEASED
- Generalize
  - Create an action plan for **PLEASED skills**
  - Problem-solve barriers
  - Commit to their plan
  - Review in next session
- Review goal sheet

Anxiety

Introduction of the topic
Anxiety Disorders encompass a large number of disorders where the primary feature is abnormal or inappropriate anxiety. Symptoms of anxiety become a problem when they occur without any recognizable trigger or when the situation does not warrant such a reaction. In other words, inappropriate anxiety is when a person's heart races, breathing increases, and muscles tense without any reason for them to do so. Studies indicate that up to 50% of individuals diagnosed with chronic pain will also meet the *DSM-V* diagnostic criteria for anxiety.

Generalized Anxiety Disorder (GAD)
The main feature of GAD is excessive and pervasive worry about many everyday life events. This worry is difficult to control, persists for more than 6 months and interferes with daily functioning.
   Other symptoms may include:

- muscle tension, aches or soreness
- feeling on edge or experiencing restlessness
- fatigue
- irritability
- difficulty concentrating
- poor sleep

The intensity, duration, or frequency of the anxiety and worry is far out of propor-
tion to the actual likelihood or impact of the feared event. The person finds it difficult
to keep worrisome thoughts from interfering with attention to tasks and has difficulty
stopping the worry. Adults with Generalized Anxiety Disorder often worry about
everyday, routine life circumstances such as possible job responsibilities, finances, the
health of family members, misfortune to their children, or minor matters (such as
household chores, car repairs, or being late for appointments). Children with Generalized Anxiety Disorder tend to worry excessively about their competence or the
quality of their performance. During the course of the disorder, the focus of worry
may shift from one concern to another.

Associated with muscle tension, there may be trembling, twitching, feeling shaky,
and muscle aches or soreness. Many individuals with Generalized Anxiety Disorder
also experience somatic symptoms (e.g., sweating, nausea, or diarrhea) and an exaggerated startle response. Symptoms of autonomic hyperarousal (e.g., accelerated
heart rate, shortness of breath, dizziness) are less prominent in Generalized Anxiety
Disorder than in other Anxiety Disorders, such as Panic Disorder and Posttraumatic
Stress Disorder. Depressive symptoms are also common.

Panic attack and panic disorder

A panic attack is characterized by four or more of the following symptoms:

1. palpitations, pounding heart, or accelerated heart rate
2. sweating
3. trembling or shaking
4. sensations of shortness of breath or smothering
5. feeling of choking
6. chest pain or discomfort
7. nausea or abdominal distress
8. feeling dizzy, unsteady, lightheaded, or faint
9. feelings of unreality (derealization) or being detached from oneself
   (depersonalization)
10. fear of losing control or going crazy
11. fear of dying
12. numbness or tingling sensations (paresthesias)
13. chills or hot flushes

Panic disorder

The diagnostic criteria for panic disorder are defined in the *DSM-V* as follows:

Recurrent unexpected panic attacks and at least one of the attacks has been followed by 1 month (or more) of one or both of the following:

- Persistent concern or worry about additional panic attacks or their consequences
- A significant maladaptive change in behavior related to the attacks

Adjustment disorder

An adjustment disorder is characterized by the development of emotional or behavioral symptoms in response to an identifiable stressor (or stressors) occurring within
3 months of the onset of the stressor. A stressor is anything that causes a great deal

of stress in the individual's life. It could be a positive event, like a wedding or purchasing a new home, or a negative event, like a family member's death, the breakup of an important relationship, or loss of a job.

These symptoms or behaviors are clinically significant as evidenced by either of the following:

- marked distress that is in excess of what would be expected from exposure to the stressor
- significant impairment in social, occupational or educational functioning

The stress-related disturbance does not meet the criteria for another specific mental disorder. Once the stressor (or its consequences) has ended, the symptoms do not persist for more than an additional 6 months. By definition, if your feelings related to the event last longer than 6 months, it will no longer qualify for an adjustment disorder diagnosis.

An adjustment disorder can occur at any time during an individual's life and there is no difference in the frequency of this disorder between males and females. Adjustment disorders are often diagnosed when it is not clear whether the individual meets the criteria for a more severe disorder, or when the actual diagnosis is uncertain. This diagnosis often gives the clinician time to further evaluate the individual during additional therapy sessions.

Teaching skills (T)

The set of suggested skills to teach in this session is designed to increase the individual's ability to cope with anxiety in a more effective manner.

The first set of suggested skills to use is designed to reduce high levels of distress. These skills are referred to as "gateway" skills. They can be used to create a path out of high levels of distress where other skills may not be effective or easily accessible. They are designed to work on a short-term basis. These skills do not solve problems, they assist the individual to not add more distress to an already distressing situation.

Distracting the Mind – Engaging in activities that disrupt current thought patterns. This skill can be used to distract the individual from catastrophizing or ruminating. Examples of this skill include engaging in rigorous physical activity, working puzzles, or any activity that requires attention and concentration. Have individuals create their own lists of activities that involve action of the body and mind. Thought-stopping is also suggested as a skill to review in this set.

Imagery – Picturing (in your mind's eye) yourself tolerating the distress. This skill can be very effective with individuals who have excessive worry. Have the individual imagine themselves being powerful like a superhero. Have them tell a story where they are able to defeat their distress, focusing on how they were able to accomplish the feat and what powers they used. This can provide information to assist the individual to not only distract himself or herself, but can provide themes for possible problem-solving strategies.

Soothing through the Senses – Engaging the five senses to promote a feeling of peace and serenity. This skill is very effective in grounding the individual into their current experience, and serves as protection from rumination and fear. *Vision* – Looking at a peaceful scene or painting. Noticing the visual details of what is being seen. *Taste* – Slowly eating a "comfort food" and noticing how each bite touches the lips, how it feels to chew and swallow. Noticing if the food is sweet or salty, hard or soft . . . focusing on the details of the experience. *Touch* – Squeezing stress balls, using lotions, and hugging soft blankets can work well to soothe the individual. Noticing how the sun or wind feels on the skin. *Smell* – Smelling scented candles, potpourri, or anything the individual identifies as pleasurable. Lavender scents tend to be very effective. *Hearing* – Listening to soothing music that mirrors the beating of the heart, such as classical or jazz.

The second set of suggested skills to use is designed to reduce the individual's vulnerability to distress. This is done through creating healthy habits.

PLEASED (PL) – Self-care skills promote well-being and reduce emotional vulnerability.

Physical health – Taking medicines as prescribed, following medical protocols, and making appointments (and attending them) when necessary.
List resources and barriers – Create a list of strengths and resources for each area of this skill. Create a list of barriers for potential problem-solving in session.
Eat balanced meals – Eat three balanced meals plus healthy snacks throughout the day. Consult your doctor or a dietician before starting a structured meal plan.
Avoid drugs and alcohol – There are many risks associated with using drugs and alcohol. Use may lead to heightened painful emotions, decreased stability, and decreased abilities to function on a daily basis.
Sleep – Healthy sleep is a must! Most individuals need between 7 and 10 hours of sleep each day.
Exercise – Exercise a minimum of 20 minutes three to five times weekly. Modify exercises to meet your physical abilities.
Daily – Practice these skills every day to create healthy habits.

Applying skills and concepts (A)

- Introduce/discuss the homework assignment on **PLEASED skills**
- Review homework from previous session
- Problem-solve barriers to this process

Generalizing skills and concepts (G)

- Problem-solve barriers to creating a plan for **PLEASED skills**
- Modify the individual's **SIP Form** to include the skills mentioned in this session

Notes to clinicians and individuals

- Anxiety has many symptoms that mirror physical conditions (hyperthyroidism) so it is important to provide psychoeducation to individuals and their support systems.

- Anxiety symptoms tend to rise and fall like a wave. The key is to identify the triggers and have a coping plan that is based in reality.
- New skills may take time to be effective. Practice skills in times of low distress to gain practice with each skill for when it is needed the most.
- It is natural to have distress in life; it is ineffective to make it worse by being unskillful. This leads to suffering, not pain.
- It is important to review the skills from the "depression" session since many of the skills will work with different forms of emotional pain.
- Identify, validate, and reinforce small changes. They are building blocks for success.
- It is important to review the diagnostic criteria for mental health disorders with individuals. Many have been diagnosed and have not had an explanation as to why.

Psychological Curriculum

Session focus: First step toward change

TAG
Teach – Apply – Generalize

- The goal of this session is to
  - Learn coping skills to improve the individual's functioning in therapy, treatment, and life
- What to discuss:
  - Exploring the sense of "being stuck"
  - Introduce 7 barriers to effective functioning
    - Thoughts
    - Feelings
    - Behaviors
    - Attitudes
    - Expectations
    - Beliefs
    - Anticipated outcomes
- Skills to teach
  - Just Noticeable Change
- Generalize
  - Create an action plan for **First Step Toward Change**
  - Problem-solve barriers
  - Commit to their plan
  - Review in next session
- Review goal sheet

First step toward change

Introduction of the topic
It is anticipated that all individuals will feel "stuck" at some point in the course of their treatment. This session is designed to lead a discussion on common points that typically present as barriers to effective functioning and positive change. The goal is to focus the individual on the presenting problem, and then introduce the skill of **Just Noticeable Change (JNC)** to refocus their efforts toward positive change. This session is highly interactive, dynamic, and requires a high degree of participation.

Barriers to effective functioning
Thoughts "How do our thoughts get in the way of doing what needs to be done?"

The "I don't know" response. This can be reframed into two themes. The first theme is not knowing HOW to do something. Validate the individual's experience and focus the individual back to skills they have learned. Identify the individual's strengths, problem-solve how the strengths can be applied to the current barrier, and create a plan of action that involves a clear commitment to skill use. The second theme is not WANTING to do something. Validation can also be an effective strategy to use in this situation. Validate the feeling of being stuck and not wanting to change things. Give the individual permission to stay stuck, and let them know you are ready to assist them when they are ready to reengage in the change process. Time and patience are key components to this strategy.

Feelings "How do our feelings get in the way of doing what needs to be done?" Emotions can present as powerful barriers. Emotional distress typically forces the individual to be reactive and at times desperate. Safety is always the first priority. Once safety has been addressed, prioritize emotional stability. Individuals typically present with one or two primary emotions that affect their functioning. Assist the individual in prioritizing their emotions. Identify what they are already doing to cope. Separate their efforts into short-term (the next 24 hours) needs and strategies, mid-term (the next two weeks) needs and strategies, and long-term (two weeks and beyond) needs and strategies. Evaluate the effectiveness of their efforts to cope with distress. Modify their existing plan to focus on skills application.

Behaviors "How do our actions (behaviors) get in the way of doing what needs to be done?" An individual's behavior is present because it meets needs, it has been reinforced, and it may be resistant to change. Problems with behaviors can be separated into two categories. The individual may be engaging in behaviors designed to get what they want instead of what they need. A need is a something an individual requires to build and maintain their functioning. It is highly valued. A want or desire is a luxury for the individual that can improve their quality of life. Wants and desires seldom have a direct impact on functioning. It is important to identify and separate behaviors into these categories. Once behavioral patterns emerge, the individual may be ready to explore which behaviors need to be reinforced, and which behaviors need to be modified. Contingency management is a key concept in this strategy.

Attitudes "How do our attitudes get in the way of doing what needs to be done?" Attitudes refer to how we mentally approach a situation or life in general. An individual's attitude has a direct influence on how they approach a situation. Attitudes do change over time, but change is typically quite slow. Attitudes develop through life experiences. They are modified through an individual's interactions with themselves, others, and their environment. A key aspect of working with attitudes is to explore whether the individual's current attitude is actually effective for them, others, and their environment. Positive attitudes lead to self-empowerment, healthy relationships, and effective interactions within systems (medical, psychological, legal, etc.). Common examples of attitudes include optimism, pessimism, willingness, and willfulness.

Optimism – Interpreting and approaching situations in a positive manner
Pessimism – Interpreting and approaching situations in a negative manner

Psychological Curriculum

Willing – Being quick to act or respond
Willful – Being intentionally self-willed or stubborn

Expectations   "How do expectations get in the way of doing what needs to be done?"
Expectations can be separated into two categories. The first is what an individual expects of themselves, and is a very important concept to explore. Expecting to be perfect and without fault is a common theme. There is no acceptable option other than success. There is no room for trying or following a process. It either is or it is not. This does not translate well to reality and daily functioning. This can also be seen in individuals who are making positive changes in their lives and begin to fear that they cannot maintain the change. If an individual expects to fail or relapse, they tend to act in ways to make that their reality. The second category is what the individual perceives to be the expectations of others. If the perception is that others expect them to be perfect in their change process, any deviation from their anticipated path is viewed as failure. They can never live up to the expectations of others. If an individual experiences a positive change in functioning that others have been waiting for, they project their fears onto others and then require themselves to be perfect in response. It is a pattern that is designed to fail.

Beliefs   "How do our beliefs get in the way of doing what needs to be done?"
A belief is something that an individual thinks is true. All individuals have beliefs and it is common for beliefs to change over time. This typically happens when something that is accepted as being true is altered due to the emergence of new information. When there is an acceptable amount of proof, the "new" truth is accepted and the "old" truth is rejected. This may be clearer through an example. An individual believes that they are not capable of changing. They state that they are too stuck in their ways, too old, or cite instances where they do the same thing repeatedly. They make their statements with conviction and believe it to be true for them. It is very effective to validate that they believe this to be true. If the individual is open to challenge, this can be done through a few simple steps.

1. Identify the belief – I am not capable of change
2. Identify the extreme stance – not capable
3. Find the kernel of truth – Change is a natural part of life or few things never change
4. Identify the challenge – Change is difficult
5. Restate the new belief – Change is hard for me

Anticipated outcomes   "How does what we anticipate happening get in the way of doing what needs to be done?"
The field of psychology studies human behavior and experience. It is commonly accepted after decades of study that human behavior cannot be predicted with a high degree of certainty and accuracy. What an individual anticipates as an outcome of their actions has a potentially large impact on their behavior. If the anticipated action

does not potentially lead to a favorable result, the individual may chose not to act. The key point is that the future is unpredictable and that our actions do not always create a predictable course or path.

Teaching skills (T)

The suggested skill to teach in this session is designed to increase the individual's ability to change their behavior or approach to situations.

Just Noticeable Change (JNC) – Engaging in a behavior that leads to a change in focus or direction. This is a "baby-steps" skill. JNC allows for taking a first step toward change. It is a short-term skill designed to change the individual's "threshold" of experience. This helps the individual to identify that small steps can have a big impact concerning the process of change.

Applying skills and concepts (A)

- Introduce/discuss the homework assignment on **First Step Toward Change**
- Review homework from previous session
- Problem-solve barriers to this process

Generalizing skills and concepts (G)

- Problem-solve barriers to creating an action plan for **First Step Toward Change**
- Assign homework on the individual's action plan

Notes to clinicians and individuals

- The topics covered in this session tend to be long-standing aspects of each individual's functioning. The goal is to identify their current barriers and create an action plan to take a first step toward positive change.
- A humorous fictitious example illustrates contrasts in attitudes and anticipated outcomes: A researcher is studying the impact of attitude on children's behaviors. One child is identified as being optimistic, and another as being pessimistic. The researcher takes the pessimistic child into a room with bright lights and tons of toys. He tells the child to do whatever, to play with as many toys as he wants and that he will return for the child in one hour. He leaves the room and watches the child through a one-way mirror. The child sits in the middle of the floor doing nothing. The researcher enters the room after one hour and asks the child why he did not play with any of the toys. The child states that he knew he would have to stop playing after an hour so "why start?" The researcher then takes the optimistic child and puts him in a dark room in the basement. In the center of the room there is a huge pile of horse manure. He tells the child he will return in one hour and shuts the door. He returns after an hour and opens the door. The child is standing in the middle of the pile throwing manure all over the room. The researcher asks the child what he is

doing. The child states, "With all of this manure – there must be a pony here somewhere!"

• Small steps can lead to large results. Consider the butterfly effect. If a butterfly flaps its wings in China, would it have an effect on the weather patterns in London? The obvious answer is no, but since every action has an effect on other probabilities . . . the implications are infinite.

Session focus: Anger management

TAG
Teach – Apply – Generalize

- The goal of this session is to
  - Identify signs and symptoms of anger
  - Learn coping skills to improve the individual's functioning in the area of anger management
- What to discuss:
  - Anger
  - Functions of anger
- Skills to teach
  - **Beliefs about Anger, Managing Conflict**
  - Imagery, Soothing through the Senses
  - Dear Man, Give
- Generalize
  - Create an action plan for **Beliefs about Anger** and **Managing Conflict**
  - Problem-solve barriers
  - Commit to their plan
  - Review in next session
- Review goal sheet

Anger management

Introduction of the topic
Anger may be defined as a normal emotion that involves a strong uncomfortable and emotional response to a perceived provocation. This definition indicates that anger is a normal emotion. Anger does not feel good to experience. Anger is also a response to a perceived trigger or event that requires action. Anger is a primary target for treatment in over 50% of the chronic pain and comorbid mental health population. It is common for individuals to respond with anger to their pain and mental health concerns. It is important to identify that anger can serve both positive and destructive functions.

Functions of anger
Anger can be viewed as a protective response to a perceived threat. Anger may help the individual respond to a situation where their safety is at risk. A useful distinction between positive and negative aspects of anger is to note the difference between the emotional state that is labeled as angry, and the negative expression of that angry state, which might be termed aggression (Gottman & Levenson, 1992; Novaco, 1983). This indicates that although anger may serve as an appropriate response to a perceived threat, it is not the same as aggression, which is acting on the emotional state of anger when there is a misperception of a threat or when no threat is present. Individuals coping with chronic conditions often respond to

situations with misplaced anger or aggression. Examples of this may include acting on fears that something will be taken away from them or that further loss will be experienced (protection), anger responses directed toward the initial loss or change in functioning (being wronged/entitled), a style of communication (frustration and entitlement), and using anger responses to meet their own needs (intimidation).

Teaching skills (T)

The suggested skills to teach in this session are designed to increase the individual's ability to cope with anger. This can be approached in a stepwise and sequential manner.

1. Discuss the functions of anger. How aware is each individual about the roles and functions that anger plays in their lives? Are their responses effective for themselves and others? Are there healthier alternatives to situations that are not working for them or others?
2. Focus the individual on how anger builds in their lives. Once triggers and patterns are identified, separate the responses into two categories – internal and external. The internal category is reserved for situations where the individual is experiencing potential errors in perception or judgment. The external category is reserved for situations where anger serves as a useful signal that a problem needs to be addressed and resolved.
3. Assign appropriate homework worksheet – **Beliefs about Anger** or **Managing Conflict**.

The second set of suggested skills to teach is designed to provide self-soothing and relaxation training.

Imagery – Picturing (in your mind's eye) yourself tolerating the distress. This skill can be very effective with individuals who have excessive worry. Have the individual imagine that they are being powerful like a superhero. Have them tell a story where they are able to defeat their distress, focusing on how they were able to accomplish the feat and what powers they used. This can provide information to assist the individual to not only distract himself or herself, but can provide themes for possible problem-solving strategies.

Soothing through the senses – Engaging the five senses to promote a feeling of peace and serenity. This skill is very effective in grounding the individual into their current experience, and serves as protection from rumination and fear. *Vision* – Looking at a peaceful scene or painting. Noticing the visual details of what is being seen. *Taste* – Slowly eating a "comfort food" and noticing how each bite touches the lips, how it feels to chew and swallow. Noticing if the food is sweet or salty, hard or soft . . . focusing on the details of the experience. *Touch* – Squeezing stress balls, using lotions, and hugging soft blankets can work well to soothe the individual. Noticing how the sun or wind feels on the skin. *Smell* – Smelling scented candles, potpourri, or anything the individual identifies as pleasurable. Lavender scents tend to be very effective. *Hearing* – Listening to soothing music that mirrors the beating of the heart, such as classical or jazz.

Monitored breathing exercises – Having individuals attempt to slow their breathing to the rate of 6 breaths per minute.

Progressive muscle relaxation is another very effective calming technique.

Guided imagery is also a very effective calming technique.

The third set of suggested skills to teach is designed to assist the individual to manage conflict more effectively. This can be done by preparing the individual for potential conflict (Homework Assignment: **Managing Conflict**) and teaching the interpersonal effectiveness skills of **DEAR MAN (DM)** and **GIVE (G)**.

DEAR MAN

Describe – Use **Observe** and **Describe** to summarize the situation and identify the facts that support the request or reason for setting a limit or boundary.

Express – Share your beliefs or opinions when relevant or required.

Assert – Ask clearly for what you want or need.

Reward – Let others know how helping you meet your wants or needs will potentially impact their situation.

Mindful – Stay focused on your request and avoid leaving the topic.

Act confident – Use an assertive tone, have confident body language, make eye contact, and stay calm.

Negotiate – Be willing to compromise to meet your wants or needs.

To apply the skill set of **DM**, the individual must first prioritize their needs. Make sure that the person you are communicating with has the capability of providing for the request. Be aware of asking the right person at the right time. Consider if it is appropriate to ask for something given the status of the current relationship. It is also important to review whether the request meets short-term wants/needs or long-term wants/needs.

GIVE

The skill set of **GIVE (G)** is designed to teach the individual to build and maintain relationships.

Gentle – Be respectful in your approach and avoid threats, demands, and attacks.

Interested – Listen to the other person and be open to the information they have to provide.

Validate – Acknowledge and attempt to understand the other person's perspective.

Easy Manner – Be political and treat others in a kind and relaxed manner.

To apply the skill set of **G**, the individual needs to balance the demands their interaction is placing on the relationship with the health of the relationship itself. The relationship may need to be nurtured or repaired before any further requests can be made.

Psychological Curriculum

Applying skills and concepts (A)

- Introduce/discuss the homework assignment on **Beliefs About Anger** and **Managing Conflict**
- Role-play anger-triggering scenarios and skills application
- Review homework from previous session
- Problem-solve barriers to this process

Generalizing skills and concepts (G)

- Have individuals share their homework with their support system and professional team
- Problem-solve barriers to effective skills applications

Notes to clinicians and individuals

- Frustration and anger are different; intensity of experience is what differentiates them.
- Many individuals may benefit from reviewing a feeling's chart to assist in identifying the different levels of anger.
- Validation and normalization are keys to engaging individuals in this process.
- Justification of action can lead to rationalization and lack of motivation for potential change.
- We all experience anger; anger only becomes a serious concern when an individual is angry too frequently, too intensely, and for too long (Novaco, 1985).

Session focus: Attending to distress

TAG
Teach – Apply – Generalize

- The goal of this session is to
  - Gain insight and information about the effects of attention and concentration applied to pain management
  - Learn coping skills to improve functioning in the areas of attention and concentration
- What to discuss:
  - Focusing on distress
  - Thinking about distress
  - Acting on Distress
- Skills to teach
  - Distract with ACCEPTS, Turning the Mind
  - Behavioral Mapping, Event Scheduling, Modifying Activities
- Generalize
  - Create an action plan for **Attributions**
  - Problem-solve barriers
  - Review in next session
- Review goal sheet

Attending to distress

Introduction of the topic
Individuals experiencing physical pain and emotional distress require a lot of time, effort, and energy in order to cope effectively. Individuals may actually make their distress worse by focusing their attention and concentration on the distress. The more an individual focuses on their distress, the more likely they are to compromise their functioning. This is demonstrated through what the individual focuses on, thinks, and does.

Focusing on distress
Focusing on distress is natural for individuals. Pain (whether it is physical or psychological) is an alarm that serves as a protective mechanism. Pain tells the individual that something is causing harm. An example of this is when we place a finger on a hot stove. The natural reaction is to quickly remove the finger from the stove. No thought is required to act. The nervous system is designed to send pain messages to the brain that trigger an automatic response – removal of the finger from the stove. This indicates that pain can serve as a messenger to protect from harm. It also indicates that we act in automatic ways to pain (escape and avoid). One of the issues is that this is a normal response to acute pain or injury. When an individual experiences pain on a daily basis the pain is no longer classified as acute, it is classified as chronic. This changes how the individual experiences the pain. The body is no longer sending the same pain messages that direct the individual's attention in the same manner and,

as a result, behaviors are no longer hard-wired (automatic), but are learned. This changes how the individual responds with coping strategies. If the individual is able to attend to the pain when it is needed, and focus elsewhere when they are making things worse, their experience of pain can be changed.

When the distress is psychological (emotional), a natural response is for the individual to focus on the negative aspects of the distress. When an individual is depressed, they may focus on the sadness, crying, isolation, and emptiness. This reinforces the experience of the distress by attending to it without acting on potential change. Unknowingly they are practicing their symptoms.

Thinking about distress

What we think affects what we do. Many individuals associate distress with control. The individual is attempting to gain cognitive control by finding a cause. This process is an attempt to find order and predictability by explaining and understanding the causes behind behaviors and situations that occur. In a sense, this is the process of how people make sense of their world; what cause and effect inferences they make about the behaviors of others and themselves. When an individual makes inferences (going beyond the information that is present), there is risk of making errors. Many individuals fear physical activity because it may cause pain. It is common to have physical discomfort when a workout routine is first started. Muscles that have not been stretched properly or used in a similar fashion become sore. There may be stiffness, soreness, or even a dull ache stemming from the new activity. This increase in discomfort may be associated with similar experiences that indicate that a flare-up may be experienced. This is not only common, but also predictable. If the individual attributes the increase in physical discomfort from working out to a possible pain trigger, the workout will be avoided out of fear of causing further pain and damage. This fear does not match the reality of the situation. A healthy behavior is then avoided because the individual made an error in associating discomfort with fearing injury. This example demonstrates that attributions and inferences have a direct impact on behaviors and activities. Remember that hurt does not always equate to harm.

When the distress is psychological (emotional), a natural response is for the individual to attribute the distress to their experiences of demoralization and loss of hope. If they blame themselves or those around them for the distress they are experiencing they increase the risk of confirming that there is some character defect in themselves or others and that the pattern will continually repeat itself. If an individual feels unsupported, they may view others as not caring or that relationships are no longer acceptable. They may be dismissive of others' attempts to support them if they are trying to prove that they are unsupported.

Acting on distress

Many individuals associate pain with the need to escape, avoid, or alter their experience. This pattern of behavior leads to extremes that do not adapt and generalize well. It is common for individuals to demonstrate extremes in behaviors when they are experiencing distress. If an individual is in physical pain, they may choose to rest in an attempt to avoid making their pain worse. It may be easier to do nothing instead of doing something, in order to avoid risk. This affects physical and psychological functioning. According to the Yale Medical Group, there are problems associated with inactivity such as:

- Increased risk for cardiovascular disease and other conditions
- Greater risk of developing high blood pressure
- Increased feelings of anxiety and depression
- Increased risk of certain cancers
- Studies indicate that physically active people are less likely to develop coronary heart disease than those who are inactive – even after the researchers accounted for smoking, alcohol use, and diet.
- Physically active overweight or obese people significantly reduce their risk for disease with physical activity.

Teaching skills (T)

The suggested skills to teach in this session are designed to increase the individual's ability to cope more effectively with physical and psychological pain through distraction skills.

Attention diversion skills – **Distract with ACCEPTS** and **Turning the Mind.**
Distract with ACCEPTS – Accept distress to effectively apply distraction skills.
Activities – Activities assist in decreasing distress and can create positive emotions. Plan activities and do something each day. Doing something is often better than doing nothing. Create an activities list of things you enjoy doing to promote a more active and healthy approach to coping with distress.
Contributing – Do something for someone else. Take a break from your own distress by engaging in others' lives in a positive manner. Smiling, volunteering support or assistance, and listening are all examples of this skill.
Comparisons – Compare your current situation to a time where you were less skillful and less effective. This can provide perspective to your current situation. You can also compare your situation to that of someone who has it worse than you. Validate your experience as you search for healthy perspectives.
Emotions – Engage in activities or thoughts that create emotions that are different from the painful ones you are currently experiencing.
Push Away – Mentally put the distress in a box on a shelf behind a locked door. Take a break from it now with the intention of addressing the issue at a safe point in the future.
Thoughts – Engage in activities that lead to different thoughts. Read a book or magazine, work a puzzle, or count to 100.
Sensations – Stimulate sensations that are safe to engage in.

Turning the Mind – Continually refocusing your attention and concentration away from the distress to the distraction activity. This may need to be done continually to be effective.

The second set of suggested skills to teach in this session is designed to increase the individual's ability to cope more effectively with physical and psychological pain by challenging ineffective thought patterns.

Inaccuracies in attribution lead to misplaced blame and blind individuals to other potential causes. According to Harold Kelley (1973), it is important to review the four rules of logic when attributing cause to an individual or a situation to avoid cognitive errors. The homework assignment on **Attributions** will provide an example of this concept that is more accessible, but it is important for the reader to understand the basic principles.

1. **Covariation (relating)** – If a behavior or object is always present when another behavior or object is present they correlate, they do not cause each other to exist. An individual leaves their apartment or house at the same time each day to take a walk in the park. If a neighbor leaves at the exact same time each day to go to work, neither is causing the other to leave. They happen to have similar schedules.

2. **Extremity (intensity)** – The more extreme the effect of a behavior, the more likely we are to make internal attributions. If an individual becomes angry and starts an argument that sends others running, they are more likely to consider themselves to be an angry person, not someone who is experiencing the emotion of anger.

3. **Discounting (dismissing)** – The more you know about environmental conditions surrounding a behavior, the less likely you are to make internal attributions. If an individual knows that their doctor is typically busy and has difficulty scheduling appointments, they are less likely to blame themselves when scheduling difficulties occur.

4. **Augmentation (increasing)** – Motivation is increased if a barrier is experienced and overcome. If an individual fears holding their child, but does so even when there is a mild increase in pain, they are more prone to hold their child again even when fear is present.

Consider the covariation of three factors when making attributions:

- **Distinctiveness of the entity** – The behavior only occurs when the entity is present (HIGH DISTINCTIVENESS). Jan is petting a dog, does she pet all dogs (LOW DISTINCTIVENESS) or only that dog? The more specific the behavior is to this one entity the less it tells us about Jan.
- **Consensus** – Do most others respond similarly? If most others respond the same way to this entity (petting), then there is HIGH CONSENSUS. If most others do not respond this way to this entity there is LOW CONSENSUS.
- **Consistency** – Does Jan act this way in the presence of this entity most of the time (HIGH CONSISTENCY) or only some of the time (LOW CONSISTENCY)?

High Distinctiveness, High Consensus, and High Consistency leads to an External attribution; Low distinctiveness, Low Consensus, and Low Consistency leads to an internal attribution.

The third sets of suggested skills to teach in this session are designed to increase the individual's ability to cope more effectively with physical and psychological pain through activity modification. When experiencing distress it is important to modify or change behaviors. These skills can be applied to both physical and psychological distress. The examples provided here target physical distress.

Behavioral mapping

It is important for the individual to recognize that certain activities lead to either an increase or a decrease in pain. The Pain Scale (See Chapter 4) will be used to establish the individual's daily routine and the role of pain in their lives. The individual is to track their activities throughout the day, how they attempted to cope, levels of pain pre/post intervention, and the location or source of their pain. This form is to be completed daily and reviewed in the second section of the program day.

Event scheduling

It is important to plan and prepare for events that may present barriers to effective functioning. The Skills Implementation Plan (SIP) form is designed to prepare the individual for anticipated activities. The form can be used to identify stressful events and create a concrete skills-based plan to promote effective coping. The individual is to complete the plan early in treatment and modify the plan as they learn and apply coping skills throughout the course of the program. It is common to have individuals identify attempts to cope with stressful situations through a wide variety of strategies. The variations in coping may be categorized into three main areas: fight, flight, and freeze, which are covered in the next section.

Modifying activities

Many individuals struggle with modifying activities. A key point of discussion is to review frequency (F) of the activity, intensity (I) of engagement, and duration (D) of involvement. Introduce the concept of altering aspects of FID through attempts at self-regulation and pacing strategies.

"Fight" is a common coping response that may be defined as: continuing to participate in an activity until its completion regardless of the pain that is experienced or produced. Many individuals tend to cope with events by "powering-through." They tend to disregard their pain triggers and continue with the activity.

"Flight" is a common coping response that may be defined as disengaging from an activity that begins to trigger a pain response. This may be very healthy at times, but may also lead to stopping an activity out of fear that a pain response may happen. This concept also includes disengaging from an activity in the anticipation that pain may be triggered.

"Freeze" is a common coping response that may be defined as avoiding any activity that may lead to a pain response. Many individuals choose to avoid activities that have no history of causing pain out of fear that pain may occur, so it is safer to avoid the entire situation.

It is important to introduce a "Behavior Chain" to assist the individual in identifying their responses to activities that may or may not affect their pain levels. This allows for review of the antecedents, the response of the individual, and the generation of behavioral alternatives that target increases in adaptive functioning.

Applying skills and concepts (A)

- Introduce/discuss the homework assignment on **Attributions**
- Review homework from previous session
- Problem-solve barriers to this process

Generalizing skills and concepts (G)

- Problem-solve barriers to creating an action plan for **Attributions**
- Assign homework on the individual's action plan

Notes to clinicians and individuals

- It is important to note that in Kelley's examination of Attribution Theory he covered the concept in depth. The reader needs to have a working knowledge of this theory to understand the details of the homework and the rationale for the work itself.
- When pain is attended to, the experience of the pain is potentially changed. This is very similar to how biofeedback works. Biofeedback is simply feedback (or information) about your biological functions. It works by detecting small changes in your body and providing you with visual information of these changes – the information is "fed back" to you. When you see this information, you can then go through a "trial and error" strategy where you learn to control your biological response.
- This session may need extended time to review with the individual. There are multiple issues to cover and extended sets of skills. Take your time and target what is most relevant to each individual.
- Be flexible and open to exploring issues and challenges. This session covers attention and concentration, thought process, and action all targeting physical and psychological distress. Lead with validation and pacing of the material.

Session focus: Meaning and pain

TAG
Teach – Apply – Generalize

- The goal of this session is to
  - Learn coping skills to improve the individual's functioning in the areas of finding meaning and increasing hope
- What to discuss:
  - Meaning and pain
  - Physical
  - Social
  - Psychological
  - Spiritual
- Skills to teach
  - Radical Acceptance
  - Practical Acceptance
  - Practical Change
  - Radical Change
  - Just Noticeable Change
- Generalize
  - Create an action plan for **Finding Meaning and Purpose**
  - Problem-solve barriers
  - Commit to their plan
  - Review in next session
- Review goal sheet

Meaning and pain

Introduction of the topic

All individuals experience some degree of pain in their lives. Pain can take many forms including physical, social, psychological, and spiritual. There is a form of pain that is termed "existential pain" which can be difficult to define. One definition is that an individual experiences suffering with no clear connection to physical pain. "Existential pain" is mostly used as a metaphor for suffering, but also is seen as a clinically important factor that may reinforce existing physical pain or even be the primary cause of pain . . . (Strang, Strang, Hultborn, & Arner, 2004). Different aspects of suffering may be present which include guilt, spiritual connection, and the idea that living is painful. Depression, anxiety, and anger are also closely associated with the concept of "Existential pain." It is important to explore the role of meaning when we experience pain. If individuals can find meaning and purpose in relation to their pain, they may be able to reduce their suffering and distress. "Existential pain" may be separated into four categories including physical, social, psychological, and spiritual.

Physical

It may be viewed that individuals first relate to their physical environment, which includes their awareness of their physical pain. When pain is present, it affects functioning. There may be limitations that are experienced, changes in abilities, financial problems, and increased risk of injury or illness.

Social

Humans are social beings. Individuals relate to others in their world. This category of pain includes relationships, cultural issues, socio-economic issues, race identity, conflict with others, competition issues, and failure.

Psychological

The psychological category includes how individuals relate to themselves and have their own personal sense of identity.

Spiritual

This category includes the individual's attitude toward the unknown and how they assign meaning to experiences. This category also includes the individual's sense of connection to something larger than themselves. This is up to each individual to define.

Teaching skills (T)

The teaching in this session is designed to be done in two phases. The first phase is based on discussion. Lead a discussion on each category of "Existential pain." Explore the meaning and purpose that individuals ascribe to their experience. The homework assignment on **Finding Meaning and Purpose** will assist in facilitating this process. The goal is to identify how the individual identifies meaning and purpose for each category. Once the discussion has been completed, the clinician can introduce skills training.

A skill set to teach in this process is designed to assist the individual in accepting their current situation while acting toward change when it is needed or desired. Not accepting reality or changing the individual's responses to it actually causes them to suffer and creates a barrier to finding purpose and meaning.

Acceptance versus change

Marsha Linehan (1993a) introduced the concept of dialectics involving the needed balance of acceptance and change to assist individuals in coping more effectively with difficulties in their lives. Acceptance is the process of acknowledging something without attempting to change it. It is not the process of quitting or giving up, but rather recognizing the reality of a situation. The reality of the individual is often an effective starting point for engagement in the therapeutic process. Many individuals do not want to accept their current situation and want everything to change. This can lead to unrealistic goals and expectations. Conversely, if we accept everything we will do nothing about our current situation and the result often leads to suffering. A new set of skills will be introduced to target this key concept in treatment which includes: practical acceptance, practical change, and radical change. These skills are designed to assist in the process of setting realistic goals and guide the individual through the process of balancing acceptance and promoting healthy change.

There is a healthy balance that can be found between acceptance and change. The concept of dialectic may be defined as a commitment to the core conditions of acceptance and change. Progress is made through combining elements that are opposite to one another to create a synthesis based in reality. An example is that I may want to be free from pain (a desire for change), but right now I experience pain on a daily basis (acceptance of what is). If an individual is able to synthesize the truth of both extremes they have an increased ability to view their experience in a more realistic manner. The synthesis may involve a combination of focusing on one or more of the skills outlined in this section.

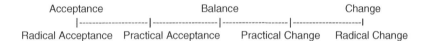

On one end of the dialectic is **Radical Acceptance** (RA). This skill may be defined as accepting reality for what it is. It is letting go of fighting or resisting one's current situation and accepting that attempts to change reality may be futile. This skill is about accepting 100% of the situation while focusing on changing how the individual copes and adapts to the situation itself.

Physical category example: An individual may need to accept that pain is a part of their everyday life and their current option is to change how they respond to this reality.

A less extreme version of this skill is **Practical Acceptance** (PA). This skill may be defined as accepting reality and understanding that controlling the situation is futile, but the individual can still influence that situation. PA encourages the individual to accept the situation for what it is while understanding they can still change aspects of the situation and how they respond to it. PA is less extreme than RA in the sense that the individual still needs to accept reality for what it is, but has not exhausted all attempts to influence (change) internal or external factors that are causing distress. The skill allows for a high degree of acceptance while encouraging appropriate action designed to promote healthy change. For example, the individual may accept 80% (most aspects that are change resistant) of the situation while targeting 20% (some aspects that can be influenced) for change.

Social category example: An individual may need to accept that pain is limiting their ability to be the kind of friend, partner, or family member that they want to be. They can still modify some of their beliefs or behaviors to change how they respond to this reality.

The next skill on the dialectic is **Practical Change** (PC). This skill may be defined as changing many aspects of a situation and needing to accept some aspects that are change resistant. PC encourages the individual to focus on action and changing the situation itself while they change how they respond. The skill allows for the promotion of a high degree of change while encouraging the acceptance that not all aspects will change. For example, the individual may target change for 80% (most aspects that can be influenced) of the situation while accepting 20% (some aspects that are change resistant).

Psychological category example: An individual may need to change many of their coping strategies to address their depression while accepting some aspects of their depression that cannot currently be changed.

The last skill on the dialectic is **Radical Change** (RC). This skill may be defined as changing all aspects of a situation because no other alternatives are acceptable. This is an extreme skill designed for application in extreme situations. RC is about changing 100% of the situation by focusing on changing how the individual copes and adapts to the situation itself.

Spiritual category example: An individual may need to change how they share their experiences with others if their current attempts are causing them to feel isolated and disconnected.

The last skill to teach in this session is designed to assist the individual in the process of balancing acceptance with change.

Just Noticeable Change (JNC) – Engaging in a behavior that leads to a change in focus or direction. This is a "baby-steps" skill. JNC allows for taking a first step toward change. It is a short-term skill designed to change the individual's "threshold" of experience. This helps the individual to identify that small steps can have a big impact concerning the process of balancing acceptance with change.

Applying skills and concepts (A)

- Review the individual's treatment plan and prioritize/modify goals and objectives as necessary
- Introduce/discuss the homework assignment on **Finding Meaning and Purpose**
- Review homework from previous session
- Problem-solve barriers to this process

Generalizing skills and concepts (G)

- Problem-solve barriers to creating an action plan for Finding Meaning and Purpose
- Assign homework on the individual's action plan

Notes to clinicians and individuals

- The topics discussed in this session are emotionally intense.
- Purpose and Meaning in life are concepts that we all struggle with.
- Many individuals may never have explored these concepts so be prepared to provide examples and be comfortable with not being able to provide answers to proposed questions.

Session focus: Stress management

TAG
Teach – Apply – Generalize

- The goal of this session is to
  - Learn coping skills to improve the individual's ability to identify stress and improve coping abilities
- What to discuss:
  - Defining stress
  - Symptoms of stress
  - Health effects of stress
- Skills to teach
  - **Stress Management Handouts**
  - Observe, Describe, Participate, Effectively
- Generalize
  - Create an action plan for **Coping with Stress Handouts**
  - Problem-solve barriers
  - Commit to their plan
  - Review in next session
- Review goal sheet

Stress management

Introduction of the topic
All individuals have some stress in their lives. This is normal and expected. It is impossible to remove all stress from any individual's life, but there are ways to decrease the negative impact on functioning. This can be done through understanding what stress is, identifying what is stressful to each individual, and learning skills to cope more effectively with stress.

Defining stress
Dr. Richard Lazarus, a prominent stress researcher, defines psychological stress as "a particular relationship between the person and the environment that is appraised by the person as taxing or exceeding his or her resources and endangering his or her well-being." This implies that different individuals can have different responses to similar stressors. It also implies that the meaning of the interaction may define if the situation is identified as stressful or not.

According to the Center for Disease Control and Prevention, stress can hit you when you least expect it – before a test, after an accident, or during conflict in a relationship. While everyone experiences stress at times, a prolonged bout of it can affect your health and ability to cope with life. That's why social support and self-care are important. They can help you see your problems in perspective . . . and the stressful feelings ease up.

Sometimes stress can be good. For instance, it can help you develop skills needed to manage potentially threatening situations in life. However, stress can be harmful when it is severe enough to make you feel overwhelmed and out of control.

Strong emotions like fear, sadness, or other symptoms of depression are normal, as long as they are temporary and don't interfere with daily activities. If these emotions last too long or cause other problems, it is a different story.

Symptoms of stress

Physical or emotional tensions are often signs of stress. They can be reactions to a situation that causes you to feel threatened or anxious. Stress can be positive (such as planning your wedding) or negative (such as dealing with the effects of a natural disaster).

According to the Centers for Disease Control and Prevention, the common reactions to a stressful event include:

- Disbelief and shock
- Tension and irritability
- Fear and anxiety about the future
- Difficulty making decisions
- Being numb to one's feelings
- Loss of interest in normal activities
- Loss of appetite
- Nightmares and recurring thoughts about the event
- Anger
- Increased use of alcohol and drugs
- Sadness and other symptoms of depression
- Feeling powerless
- Crying
- Sleep problems
- Headaches, back pains, and stomach problems
- Trouble concentrating

Health effects of stress

According to Burrows (2006), it is now considered a well-established fact that psychological stress can be a trigger or important factor in a variety of physical symptoms and disease processes. There is abundant evidence of this link in the medical literature as well as in current medical practices. For example:

- Medical research suggests that up to 90% of all illness and disease is stress related, according to the Centers for Disease Control and Prevention.
- Evidence shows chronic stress can lower immunity and make people more susceptible to infections. Conversely, stress-reduction strategies, such as meditation, relaxation, and exercise, have been shown to help reverse this effect (by increasing the number of infection-fighting T cells and feel-good chemicals called endorphins in the body, for example) and prevent disease.
- Stress has been shown to contribute to the development of heart disease and high blood pressure. As a result of those findings, most heart programs incorporate

stress management and exercise, and stress reduction now plays a very prominent role in both the treatment and prevention of cardiovascular diseases.

- Skin doctors have found that many skin conditions, such as hives and eczema, are related to stress.
- Stress is thought to be a common cause of everyday aches, pains, and health problems, such as headaches, backaches, stomachaches, diarrhea, sleep loss, and loss of sex drive. Stress also appears to stimulate appetite and contribute to weight gain.

Teaching skills (T)

The first suggested sets of skills to teach are designed to increase the individual's awareness of what is stressful to them, and to assess whether their current coping strategies are effective.

Observe – Noticing one's experience
Describe – The process of putting words on one's experience
Participate – Noting what the individual is doing to cope with the current situation and how present they are in the process

When these skills are used in combination or in a linear fashion, they provide a process to recognize patterns of thoughts and behaviors. They can be used to identify how an individual interprets, reacts, and attempts to cope with an event. This promotes increased awareness of how an individual typically responds to events.

This set of skills can be used to identify where the individual is in terms of current levels of stress, triggers for stress, and how they are currently attempting to cope with their stress. Once this has been completed, they can apply the skill of **Effectively**.

Effectively – Needs are being met in a safe and healthy manner

This skill is important to teach and review when identifying whether the individual's current functioning is optimal or acceptable. Observe, describe, and participate provides information about patterns involving stress and current coping efforts. Effectively provides information about how effective the individual is being. If what they are doing meets their needs in a safe and healthy manner, continue the plan. If what they are currently doing does not meet these criteria, have the individual select and practice a stress management technique that they believe may be effective for them.

Applying skills and concepts (A)

- Lead and discuss the exercises from the **Stress Management Handouts**
- Review homework from previous session
- Problem-solve barriers to this process

Generalizing skills and concepts (G)

- Problem-solve barriers to creating an action plan for the implementation of one of the **Stress Management Handouts**
- Assign homework on the individual's action plan

Psychological Curriculum

Notes to clinicians and individuals

- Caution individuals to avoid comparing their stress levels and reactions to those of others. This is typically done in a negative and ineffective manner.
- Each individual reacts to stress differently, it is not about being "right" or "wrong," it is finding what works.
- Remember that individuals are doing the best that they can, considering their current resources.
- Skills add more "tools" to their "tool belt."
- Interpretations of events are a key to understanding the impact of stressful events.
- Remember to focus on effective skills application, remind individuals to take in the beauty that life has to offer, and most importantly – breathe.
- Stress management handouts were adapted by B. Holtberg from Kabat-Zinn's work (1991).

Session focus: Defense mechanisms and coping styles

TAG
Teach – Apply – Generalize

- The goal of this session is to
  - Gain insight and information about common defense mechanisms and coping strategies applied to pain management
  - Learn coping skills to improve patient functioning in the areas of common defense mechanisms
- What to discuss:
  - Define defense mechanisms
  - Healthy use
  - Unhealthy use
- Skills to teach
  - Observe
  - Describe
  - Participate
  - Effectively
- Generalize
  - Create an action plan for **Defense Mechanisms and Coping Styles**
  - Problem-solve barriers
  - Commit to their plan
  - Review in next session
- Review goal sheet

Defense mechanisms and coping styles: DSM-IV-TR (1994)

Introduction of the topic

Defense mechanism is a term that professionals use to describe how an individual responds to situations that are stressful or threatening. Most people have heard the phrases "he is in denial" or she is "acting out." These are common phrases used to explain how individuals cope with distress. Defense mechanisms are not "good" or "bad." They are coping styles that serve the function of protection and which allow many individuals to function in a healthy and competent manner. There are both healthy and unhealthy behaviors associated with each style, as shown below. Difficulties happen when defense mechanisms are overused to avoid dealing with situations, facing problems, or experiencing emotions. The following table shows the healthy and unhealthy sides of typical coping styles.

Coping Style	*Healthy behavior*	*Unhealthy behavior*
Acting out – The individual copes with stress by engaging in actions rather than reflections or feelings	Feeling high levels of distress and turning energy toward walking, working out, or completing tasks	Throwing temper tantrums, acting impulsively, being aggressive
Affiliation – Involves turning to other people for support	Sharing your experience with others, asking for support or validation	Having others do things for you that you can do, becoming dependent on others, losing independence
Altruism – Meeting internal needs through helping others	Feeling high levels of distress and distracting yourself by helping a friend or neighbor, volunteering your time, becoming active in the community or with an organization	Putting others' needs before your own or engaging in self-neglect
Avoidance – Refusing to deal with or encounter unpleasant objects or situations	Feeling high levels of distress and taking a break, distracting yourself for brief periods of time, doing something nice for yourself	Sticking your head in the sand, pretending things don't exist, escaping, avoiding, or altering the distress
Compensation – Overachieving in one area to compensate for failures in another	Feeling high levels of distress and turning energy toward things you do well, applying the **Building Mastery** skill, doing things to feel competent	Masking, engaging in things you do well to falsely appear competent, pretending you are doing well when you are not
Denial – Refusal to acknowledge or recognize reality. Individuals who abuse drugs or alcohol often deny that they have a problem, while victims of traumatic events may deny that the event ever occurred	Feeling high levels of distress and applying the skill **Push Away**, leaving a situation for a short period of time with a plan to return and address the distress	Leaving a situation with no plan to return or address distress, denying what is real and letting your problems build, invalidating your own experience
Devaluation – Dealing with distress by attributing exaggerated negative qualities to yourself or others	Feeling high levels of distress and applying the **Comparisons** skill to *aspects* or *objects* that are involved in order to be able to take small steps to address the situation or distress	Decreasing your self-esteem, hurting others, or minimizing the impact of the distress
Displacement – Taking out frustrations, feelings, and impulses on people or objects that are less powerful or less threatening	Feeling high levels of distress and punching a pillow, tearing a phone book, holding an ice cube in your hand	Destroying property, "kicking the dog," making those around you feel miserable

Coping Style	*Healthy behavior*	*Unhealthy behavior*
Projection – Dealing with distressing emotions or situations by falsely attributing unacceptable feelings, impulses, or thoughts to others	Feeling cool, calm, and calculating and identifying with the same qualities in others, treating others with respect when they are not being respectful toward you	Denying your own experience by placing it on others, fearing someone will leave you and blaming them for being distant, feeling frustrated and accusing others of being angry
Rationalization – Explaining an unacceptable behavior or feeling in a rational or logical manner, so avoiding the true reasons for the behavior	Feeling high levels of distress and focusing on what you are doing well, engaging in positive self-talk, riding the wave of the current emotion and reminding yourself that the distress will not last forever	Blaming others, attributing failure to the personal qualities of others, devaluing others when you feel hurt or rejected, or labeling your behavior as acceptable because others would act the same way
Regression – When confronted by stressful events, abandoning coping strategies and returning to patterns of behavior used earlier in development	Feeling high levels of distress and simplifying your life for a short period of time, engaging in the skill of **Soothing through the Senses**, asking others for support and validation, having others take care of your needs for a short period of time to get a break from your distress	Throwing temper tantrums, locking yourself in your room, becoming impulsive, acting out

Teaching skills (T)

The suggested skills to teach in this session are designed to increase the individual's ability to cope more effectively with physical and psychological distress.

Defense mechanisms meet the individual's needs, but can be ineffective, overused, or become problematic. It is important for the individual to understand when and how these mechanisms are used in times of distress. The skills of **Observe** and **Describe** can be used to identify patterns and triggers. The skills of **Participate** and **Effectively** can be used in combination to identify which coping styles are being acted on and whether they are working for the individual, others, and the systems they are a part of.

Observe – Noticing one's experience
Describe – The process of putting words on one's experience
Participate – Noting what the individual is doing to cope with the current situation and how present they are in the process

When these skills are used in combination or in a linear fashion, they provide a process to recognize patterns of thoughts and behaviors. They can be used to identify how an individual interprets, reacts, and attempts to cope with an event. This promotes increased awareness of how an individual typically responds to events.

Effectively – Needs are being met in a safe and healthy manner

This skill is important to teach and review when identifying whether the individual's current functioning is optimal or acceptable. Observe, describe, and participate provides information about patterns and where the individual is in the stages of change process. Effectively provides information about how effective the individual is being. If what they are doing meets their needs in a safe and healthy manner, continue the plan.

Applying skills and concepts (A)

- Introduce/discuss the homework assignment on **Defense Mechanisms and Coping Styles**
- Review homework from previous session
- Problem-solve barriers to this process

Generalizing skills and concepts (G)

- Problem-solve barriers to creating an action plan for **Defense Mechanisms and Coping Styles**
- Assign homework on the individual's action plan

Notes to clinicians and individuals

- We all defend ourselves when we are in distress or feel threatened in some way.
- It is important to have individuals identify 2–3 coping styles that work for them, others, and their systems (family, medical, insurance). Find reinforcers to assist the individual in building or maintaining what is working for them.
- It is important to target 2–3 coping styles that are currently ineffective and create an action plan to modify their attempts to cope in a healthy and effective manner.
- Have individuals provide examples of each defense mechanism or coping style that is effective at times and ineffective at other times. It is a valuable exercise to identify that an individual's needs have been met through their efforts while identifying the cost of such efforts on themselves, their relationships, and support systems.
- Systems may be defined as any group that the individual interacts with, such as family systems, medical systems, insurance systems, legal systems, and psychological systems.

Session focus: Stigma

TAG
Teach – Apply – Generalize

- The goal of this session is to
  - Gain insight and understanding into the effects of stigma
  - Learn coping skills to improve the individual's ability to cope effectively with stigma
- What to discuss:
  - Stigma
  - Stigma and chronic pain/mental health
  - Impact of stigma on the individual
  - Negative associations
- Skills to teach
  - Turning the Mind
  - Thought-Stopping and Positive Self-talk
  - Fast
  - Give
  - Dear Man
- Generalize
  - Create an action plan for **Challenging Stigma**
  - Problem-solve barriers
  - Commit to their plan
  - Review in next session
- Review goal sheet

Stigma

Introduction of the topic

According to the Center for Disease Control and Prevention, stigma has been defined as an attribute that is deeply discrediting. This stigmatized trait sets the bearer apart from the rest of society, bringing with it feelings of shame and isolation. Often, when a person with a stigmatized trait is unable to perform an action because of the condition, other people view the person as the problem rather than viewing the condition as the problem. More recent definitions of stigma focus on the results of stigma – the prejudice, avoidance, rejection, and discrimination directed at people believed to have an illness, disorder, or other trait perceived to be undesirable. Stigma causes needless suffering, potentially causing a person to deny symptoms, delay treatment, and refrain from daily activities. Stigma can exclude people from access to housing, employment, insurance, and appropriate medical care. Thus, stigma can interfere with prevention efforts, and examining and combating stigma is a public health priority.

Stigma and chronic pain/mental health

There is little doubt that individuals and professionals need further information and training on the treatment of chronic pain. A research panel found that typically only about 10 hours of four-year medical programs are devoted to pain and its treatment. This may further complicate the treatment of chronic pain, which has been labeled as "an invisible disability." Here are common examples of the stigmas that individuals with chronic conditions experience:

- Pain is a way to escape reality (avoidance)
- You are not tough enough (weakness)
- You are not motivated enough (resistant)
- You don't want to be fixed (broken)
- You should . . . (invalidating)
- You are living off the government (Freeloader)
- You're making yourself hurt so you can get drugs (addict)
- You are just a whiner (weakness)
- You are trying to avoid work (lazy)
- You are trying to get attention (needy)
- Your pain is not real – it's all in your head (faking)
- You're not really that badly off (catastrophizing)
- Your pain flares up at convenient times (manipulation)
- Other people are doing better than you are (minimizing)
- You are "crazy," "nuts," or "psycho" (devaluing)

Impact of stigma on the individual
According to the Substance Abuse and Mental Health Services Administration (SAMHSA) and the National Alliance on Mental Illness (NAMI), stigma leads to . . .

- Inadequate insurance coverage for mental health services
- Fear, mistrust, and violence against people living with mental illness and their families
- Family and friends turning their backs on people with mental illness
- Prejudice and discrimination
- Keeping people from getting good jobs and advancing in the workplace
- Discouraging people from getting help

Negative associations
Another impact that stigma has on the individual is the possibility of internalizing messages that they are exposed to. Consider the implications of the following saying. "If one person tells you that you have a tail, laugh and dismiss the message. If five people tell you that you have a tail, say nothing and consider the message. If ten people tell you that you have a tail, you had better turn around." If the people telling the individual that they have a tail are all experts at recognizing tails the message is probably valid and the individual may need to turn around. If the people telling the individual that they have a tail have never seen a tail before, the source of the message needs to be considered before turning around. Many people who send messages through stigma may have the best intentions, but they are probably not experts on chronic pain and mental health. The important point is that if individuals are

bombarded by half-truths and untruths, they may question their own experience and start believing in these messages. This is a significant concern that can have a direct impact on the individual's functioning and identity (and can lead to stopping medications, missing appointments, decreased self-esteem and self-worth, etc.).

Teaching skills (T)

The suggested skills to teach in this session are designed to increase the individual's ability to cope more effectively with negative messages.

The first skill set to teach in this session is **Turning the Mind (TM)**.

Turning the Mind – Continually refocusing your attention and concentration away from the distress to the distraction activity. This may need to be done continually to be effective.

When this skill is applied effectively it can assist the individual to focus their attention away from negative messages and toward their own reality and skill use. It may serve as a first line of defense against negative messages.

The second skill set to teach in this session is thought-stopping and positive self-talk (creating new tapes). These skills are designed to interrupt negative thought patterns and replace the negative messages with positive ones.

Thought-stopping – Say "STOP" when you experience automatic negative thoughts (ANTS). This breaks a negative thought cycle *for the moment* only. It may be helpful to imagine a bunch of ants running on the ground like thoughts in your head. This serves as a reminder and a distraction. Then move to the next skill of positive self-talk.

Positive Self-Talk – Replace negative messages and "old tapes that play in your head" with positive messages by creating "new tapes" that you create. Once you have stopped the negative thought cycle, identify positive messages that you can say to yourself. Practice these positive messages over and over. If negative messages have changed what you think, feel, and do, so will positive and healthy messages. We have all heard many negative messages throughout our lives, we have a choice to replace those negative messages with positive ones – and it all starts with you!

The third skill set to teach in this session is **FAST (F)**.

The skill set of **FAST (F)** is designed to teach the individual how to have self-respect and self-worth.

Fair – Be fair to yourself and others.
Apologies – Do not engage in unnecessary apologetic behavior.
Stick to values – Use your own value system as a guide for your behavior.
Truthful – Be honest and accountable to yourself and others.

When this skill is applied effectively, the individual can dismiss painful messages by relying on their own values and by treating themselves respectfully. It can also reconnect the individual to their own truth in their experiences. There is no need to apologize for what they are experiencing and know to be true for themselves.

The fourth skill set to teach in this session is **GIVE (G)**.

The skill set of **GIVE (G)** is designed to teach the individual to build and maintain relationships.

Gentle – Be respectful in your approach and avoid threats, demands, and attacks.
Interested – Listen to the other person and be open to the information they have to provide.
Validate – Acknowledge and attempt to understand the other person's perspective.
Easy Manner – Be political and treat others in a kind and relaxed manner.

This is an important skill set to apply in addressing relationships with themselves and others. The focus of this skill is to have the individual validate his or her own experience. When this skill is applied effectively, it decreases the need to rely on others for validation that they may not provide.

The fifth skill set to teach in this session is **DEAR MAN (DM)**.

Assertiveness training is a key component to setting limits and boundaries or asking for something the individual wants. The skill set of **DEAR MAN (DM)** is designed to teach the individual to increase the probability of getting their wants or needs met.

Describe – Use **Observe** and **Describe** to summarize the situation and identify the facts that support the request or reason for setting a limit or boundary.
Express – Share your beliefs or opinions when relevant or required.
Assert – Ask clearly for what you want or need.
Reward – Let others know how helping you meet your wants or needs will potentially impact their situation.
Mindful – Stay focused on your request and avoid leaving the topic.
Act confident – Use an assertive tone, have confident body language, make eye contact, and stay calm.
Negotiate – Be willing to compromise to meet your wants or needs.

To apply the skill set of **DM**, the individual must first prioritize their needs. Make sure that the person you are communicating with has the capability of providing for the request. Be aware of asking the right person at the right time. Consider if it is appropriate to ask for something given the status of the current relationship. It is also important to review whether the request meets short-term wants/needs or long-term wants/needs.

Applying skills and concepts (A)

* Introduce/discuss the homework assignment on **Challenging Stigma**
* Review homework from previous session
* Problem-solve barriers to this process

Generalizing skills and concepts (G)

* Problem-solve barriers to creating an action plan for **Challenging Stigma**
* Assign homework on the individual's action plan

Notes to clinicians and individuals

- There are extended skill sets in this session to teach and review. This allows for customizing treatment to the individual's needs.
- Stigma is a daily experience for some individuals.
- Stigma has a direct impact on thoughts, feelings, and emotions.
- Stigma can reduce motivation and compliance.
- Find ways for individuals to link and apply skills in combinations.
- The lists are designed to facilitate discussion and identify the impact of stigma on each individual.
- If the individual has active use that prevents them from participating or Dependence, they may need to be referred to primary chemical dependency (CD) treatment.

Psychological Curriculum

Session focus: Chemical abuse

TAG
Teach – Apply – Generalize

- The goal of this session is to
  - Learn coping skills to improve the individual's functioning in the area of accepting reality
  - Learn coping skills to improve the individual's functioning in the area of chemical abuse
- What to discuss:
  - Motivation to reject reality
  - Ways to escape from reality
  - Ways to avoid reality
  - Ways to alter reality
- Skills to teach
  - Distract with ACCEPTS and Turning the Mind
  - Distracting the Mind, Imagery, Soothing through Senses
  - Urge Surfing, Bridge Burning, PLEASED
- Generalize
  - Create an action plan to address **Living Life on Life's Terms**
  - Problem-solve barriers
  - Commit to their plan
  - Review in next session
- Review goal sheet

Chemical abuse

Introduction of the topic

It is important to understand the negative consequences individuals may experience when they are abusing chemicals. There may be repeated failure to fulfill major role obligations, repeated use in situations in which it is physically hazardous, multiple legal problems, and recurrent social and interpersonal problems. Individuals may also build tolerance and experience withdrawal symptoms. When an individual continues to abuse chemicals even when their quality of life is diminished, this tends to lead to a multitude of problems in many areas of their lives.

- Role obligations – problems with repeated absences or poor work performance related to substance use; substance-related absences, suspensions, or expulsions from school; neglect of children or household responsibilities.
- Physically hazardous – driving an automobile or operating a machine when impaired by substance use.
- Legal problems – arrests for substance-related disorderly conduct; DUIs.
- Social and interpersonal problems – arguments with spouse about consequences of intoxication, physical fights.

There are many reasons why individuals abuse chemicals. When individuals discuss their chemical abuse, three main themes tend to emerge. These themes are the urge to escape, avoid, and alter their current reality.

Escape
When an individual is in physical pain, psychological pain, or both, there may be urges to escape the situation or experience. When an individual's ability to cope with their current experience is beyond their threshold, urges to escape are high. Urges create very powerful motivation for change. Individuals can become desperate for temporary relief. When individuals are desperate for change their focus is purely on the relief and not the potential consequences. Urges to escape can also take a less desperate form. Urges to escape aches and frustration can also be powerful motivations to change. An important point to note is that as urges to escape become more intense, the probability of behaviors designed to act upon those urges increases.

Avoid
Avoidance is another coping strategy that can include chemical abuse. If an individual anticipates a distressing event or situation, they may engage in use to avoid the situation. This type of avoidance strategy can take many different forms. When an individual is at a social function and they are hesitant to disclose information about themselves, they may be able to avoid attending or participating through chemical use. Another example is when an individual anticipates a task will lead to an increase in pain that leads to a negative cycle, they may engage in use to break and avoid the cycle. An important point to note in this section is that an individual's pattern of use is in response to something that is anticipated, not currently being experienced.

Alter
This is a very common theme in chemical abuse. Many individuals have urges to alter their current experience, or one they anticipate to occur. When an individual is in high distress, they may experience urges to alter their current reality. This happens when individuals are about to reach, or have reached, their threshold of acceptable reality. Their attempts to cope without chemicals are not working or it is too taxing to continue. "I need a break" or "This is too much for me to take" are common statements. "Taking the edge off" is another example. This is an attempt to modify what they are currently experiencing, not an attempt to escape or avoid. These examples do not include taking medications as prescribed, but are commonly referred to as self-medicating.

Teaching skills (T)

The suggested skills to teach in this session are designed to assist the individual in coping with distress and to reduce high urges to abuse chemicals.

Attention diversion skills – **Distract with ACCEPTS** and **Turning the Mind**

Distract with ACCEPTS – Accept distress to effectively apply distraction skills.

Activities – Activities assist in decreasing distress and can create positive emotions. Plan activities and do something each day. Doing something is often better than doing nothing. Create an activities list of things you enjoy doing to promote a more active and healthy approach to coping with distress.

Contributing – Do something for someone else. Take a break from your own distress by engaging in others' lives in a positive manner. Smiling, volunteering support or assistance, and listening are all examples of this skill.

Comparisons – Compare your current situation to a time where you were less skillful and less effective. This can provide perspective to your current situation. You can also compare your situation to that of someone who has it worse than you. Validate your experience as you search for healthy perspectives.

Emotions – Engage in activities or thoughts that create emotions that are different from the painful ones you are currently experiencing.

Push Away – Mentally put the distress in a box on a shelf behind a locked door. Take a break from it now with the intention of addressing the issue at a safe point in the future.

Thoughts – Engage in activities that lead to different thoughts. Read a book or magazine, work a puzzle, or count to 100.

Sensations – Stimulate sensations that are safe to engage in.

Turning the Mind – Continually refocusing your attention and concentration away from the distress to the distraction activity. This may need to be done continually to be effective.

The second set of suggested skills to use is designed to reduce high levels of distress. These skills are referred to as "gateway" skills. They can be used to create a path out of high levels of distress where other skills may not be effective or easily accessible. They are designed to work on a short-term basis. These skills do not solve problems, they assist the individual to not add more distress to an already distressing situation.

Distracting the Mind – Engaging in activities that disrupt current thought patterns. This skill can be used to distract the individual from catastrophizing or ruminating. Examples of this skill include engaging in rigorous physical activity, working puzzles, or any activity that requires attention and concentration. Have individuals create their own lists of activities that involve action of the body and mind. Thought-stopping is also suggested as a skill to review in this set.

Imagery – Picturing (in your mind's eye) yourself tolerating the distress. This skill can be very effective with individuals who have excessive worry. Have the individual imagine themselves being powerful like a superhero. Have them tell a story where they are able to defeat their distress, focusing on how they were able to accomplish the feat and what powers they used. This can provide information to assist the individual to not only distract himself or herself, but can provide themes for possible problem-solving strategies.

Soothing through the Senses (SS) – Engaging the five senses to promote a feeling of peace and serenity. This skill is very effective in grounding the individual into their current experience, and serves as protection from rumination and fear. *Vision* – Looking at a peaceful scene or painting. Noticing the visual details of what is being seen. *Taste* – Slowly eating a "comfort food" and noticing how each bite touches the lips, how it feels to chew and swallow. Noticing if the food is sweet or salty, hard or soft . . . focusing on the details of the experience. *Touch* – Squeezing stress balls, using lotions, and hugging soft blankets can work well to soothe the individual. Noticing how the sun or wind feels on the skin. *Smell* – Smelling scented candles, potpourri, or anything the individual identifies as pleasurable. Lavender scents tend to be very effective. *Hearing* – Listening to soothing music that mirrors the beating of the heart, such as classical or jazz.

The third set of suggested skills to use is designed to assist the individual to cope more effectively with high urges to use chemicals to escape, avoid, or alter their reality.

Urge Surfing (US) – Accepting distressing urges and emotions and riding the ups and downs of the experience like a surfer rides a wave.

Pain and distress do not stay at the same levels for extended periods. We experience natural changes in intensity. It is important to remember that urges will decrease over time if the individual does not act to make them worse. Other skills may need to be applied to decrease the intensity of the distress or urges *while* this skill is being used. This skill is similar to the "pause" button on a remote. It allows the individual to stop and notice how their pain and distress levels shift over time. Their primary job at this point is to not make things worse.

Bridge Burning (BB) – Removing the means to act on potentially harmful urges.

This skill can be used to remove alcohol and drugs from immediate access in a time of crisis. The individual may need to avoid bars and associates who use chemicals until the urge reduces or is no longer a trigger for action. Changing routines typically associated with use may be helpful.

The fourth set of suggested skills to use is designed to reduce the individual's vulnerability to pain and distress. This is done through creating healthy habits over time.

PLEASED (PL) – Self-care skills promote well-being and reduce emotional vulnerability.

Physical health – Taking medicines as prescribed, following medical protocols, and making appointments (and attending them) when necessary.

List resources and barriers – Create a list of strengths and resources for each area of this skill. Create a list of barriers for potential problem-solving in session.

Eat balanced meals – Eat three balanced meals plus healthy snacks throughout the day. Consult your doctor or a dietician before starting a structured meal plan.

Avoid drugs and alcohol – There are many risks associated with using drugs and alcohol. Use may lead to heightened painful emotions, decreased stability, and decreased abilities to function on a daily basis.

Sleep – Healthy sleep is a must! Most individuals need between 7 and 10 hours of sleep each day.

Exercise – Exercise a minimum of 20 minutes three to five times weekly. Modify exercises to meet your physical abilities.

Daily – Practice these skills every day to create healthy habits.

Psychological Curriculum

Applying skills and concepts (A)

- Introduce/discuss the homework assignment on **Living Life on Life's Terms**
- Review homework from previous session
- Problem-solve barriers to this process
- Share the Alcohol abuse handout from the CDC (www.cdc.gov) as a further guide for discussion

Generalizing skills and concepts (G)

- Problem-solve barriers to creating an action plan for **Living Life on Life's Terms**
- Assign homework on the individual's action plan

Notes to clinicians and individuals

- We all experience urges that are potentially harmful to us in some manner (eating too much and feeling nauseous, overspending, driving too fast). It is what we do about our urges that either leads us to danger or promotes health.
- The skills in this session are designed to provide distraction, promote safe activity, and reduce vulnerability.
- Individuals abuse many chemicals from over-the-counter drugs to caffeine and prescription medications.
- It may be important to discuss medication sharing and passing between individuals in a group setting, waiting area, or in other areas of their lives.
- It is healthy to discuss the role of abstinence and harm-reduction.
- The reader is strongly encouraged to read more on addiction and chronic pain. Source material provided by Fishbain et al. (1992).

Session focus: Lifespan issues

TAG
Teach – Apply – Generalize

- The goal of this session is to
  - Learn coping skills to improve the individual's functioning in the areas of life-transitions
- What to discuss:
  - Healthy development
  - Ages and developmental tasks
  - Potential impact of chronic pain and mental health
- Skills to teach
  - **Master Skills Sheet**
- Generalize
  - Create an action plan for **Identifying My Developmental Tasks**
  - Create an action plan for **Working toward Healthy Development**
  - Problem-solve barriers
  - Commit to their plan
  - Review in next session
- Review goal sheet

Lifespan issues

Introduction of the topic
Many theorists in the field of psychology have identified certain tasks that adults are presented with as they age. These tasks are biological, psychological, and social in nature. There is no "right" or "wrong" way for individuals to develop. It is a process. The successful completion of these tasks at critical moments in the course of their life leads the individual to healthy functioning and increases their chances for successful completion of subsequent tasks. There are certain aspects of development that are affected by chronic pain and mental health. There may be delays in completing these tasks or an inability to find healthy resolution. This session is designed to address the common developmental tasks that most adults are faced with and provide a context for skills application to facilitate healthy growth for the individual.

Ages and developmental tasks
According to Havighurst (1972), there are certain tasks associated with age-based categories that are seen to be important to promote healthy development.

(Ages 18–30) Young adulthood   Selecting a mate. Learning to live with a partner. Starting family. Rearing children. Managing home. Getting started in occupation. Taking on civic responsibility. Finding a congenial social group.

   At this stage of development, individuals are presented with tasks that focus on connecting with others by finding a partner and raising a family, finding a group of individuals to connect with for social outlets and support, connecting to one's community, and creating a stable living situation. This can be challenging to accomplish for any individual and may be even more challenging due to the impact of physical pain and psychological distress.

(Ages 30–60) Middle age Assisting teenage children to become responsible and happy adults. Achieving adult social and civic responsibility. Reaching and maintaining satisfactory performance in one's occupational career. Developing adult leisure-time activities. Relating oneself to one's spouse as a person. Accepting and adjusting to the physiological changes of middle age. Adjusting to aging parents.

At this stage of development, individuals are presented with the tasks of raising their children, building and maintaining a career, balancing work with healthy leisure activities, continuing to build intimacy with a partner, adjusting to how the body is changing with age, and coping with parents who are facing end-of-life issues.

(60 and over) Older adulthood Adjusting to decreasing physical strength and health. Adjusting to retirement and reduced income. Adjusting to death of a spouse. Establishing an explicit affiliation with one's age group. Adopting and adapting social roles in a flexible way. Establishing satisfactory physical living arrangements.

At this stage of development, individuals are presented with the tasks of adjusting to changes in their health and physical abilities, anticipating and planning for retirement, adjusting to changes in income, connecting with others who are in similar situations, changing social contacts and roles, and modifying or finding an appropriate place to live.

Potential impact of chronic pain and mental health
When individuals are challenged with physical and psychological problems, their healthy development may be threatened. Many of the tasks that are identified in the *60 and over* category of development are actually experienced earlier. Therefore, while individuals are presented with their age-appropriate tasks of development, they also experience the additional tasks from the next stage. This creates a lot of distress for an individual who is already spending a lot of time, effort, and energy coping with their current situation. The end result is a high level of stress and multiple tasks to address that many of the individual's peers do not yet need to address. This scenario represents an acceleration in developmental tasks that the individual is seldom prepared to address.

Teaching skills (T)

The suggested skills to teach in this session are designed to assist the individual to cope more effectively with their current stage of development.

The sets of skills that can be taught in this session will be accomplished through the homework assignments. In the current session, each individual will identify what their current developmental tasks are and how they are coping with them (**Identifying My Developmental Tasks**). Once this work is completed, they will be assigned the homework of **Working toward Healthy Development**. This requires the individual to create a skills-based plan to assist them in coping more effectively. The skills to be used can be referenced from the **MASTER SKILLS SHEET** to customize the action plan to each individual.

Applying skills and concepts (A)

- Introduce/discuss the homework assignments of **Identifying My Developmental Tasks** and **Working toward Healthy Development**
- Review homework from previous session
- Problem-solve barriers to this process

Generalizing skills and concepts (G)

- Problem-solve barriers to creating an action plan for **Working toward Healthy Development**
- Assign homework on the individual's action plan

Notes to clinicians and individuals

- This session starts with identification of where individuals are stuck in their lives and encourages them to focus on the "Bigger Picture" to move forward.
- Have individuals select skills for their action plan that are designed to provide motivation and positive movement.
- Complete the **Identifying My Developmental Tasks** worksheet in session and assign the **Working toward Healthy Development** worksheet as homework.
- Remind individuals that if their focus is on the past and what they have lost, or too much on their current distress, they are not attending to current possibilities or planning for the future. This is how individuals stay "stuck" in the developmental process.
- Change is a natural process that can be both painful and liberating.

Session focus: Managing flare-ups

TAG
Teach – Apply – Generalize

- The goal of this session is to
  - ○ Identify triggering events and typical reactions
  - ○ Learn coping skills to improve the individual's functioning in the areas of fear and avoidance
- What to discuss:
  - ○ Coping with pain
  - ○ Fears of reinjury
  - ○ Negative feedback loop
- Skills to teach
  - ○ Observe, Describe, Participate
  - ○ Effectively
  - ○ Creating a Skills Implementation Plan (**SIP**)
  - ○ Behavior chain
- Generalize
  - ○ Create an action plan for **Turning Fear and Inactivity Into Action and Hope**
  - ○ Problem-solve barriers
  - ○ Commit to their plan
  - ○ Review in next session
- Review goal sheet

Managing flare-ups

Introduction of the topic

Learning how to manage physical pain involves trial-and-error learning for both the individual and the professionals involved in their care. Each individual has his or her own unique experience of pain. It may be difficult to predict when physical pain will occur or intensify. This may have a significant impact on functioning. When pain is unpredictable, many individuals choose to minimize their risk of increasing their pain. This can be accomplished by stopping an activity or not engaging in the activity at all. In the short term, this will meet many needs. Individuals are able to avoid increases in pain, they are able to rest, and they may be able to avoid unwanted tasks or physical activities. When this is a long-term strategy, it leads to a variety of difficulties including fear, anxiety, inactivity, decreased muscle tone, weight gain, loss of physical functioning, and potentially increased physical distress (due to inactivity). Since avoiding pain is a natural and understandable response, it is important to identify when this method of coping is effective, and when other strategies and behaviors are needed. There are two main barriers for many individuals – fears of reinjury and negative cycling.

Fears of reinjury

Many individuals have strong fears of reinjury. This fear may be reinforced because of a history of reinjury. If an individual acted beyond their limitations or experienced further physical trauma, they are acting on a negative reinforcement schedule to avoid similar situations in the future. Behaviors are negatively reinforced when they allow the individual to escape from aversive stimuli that are already present or when they allow the individual to avoid the aversive stimuli before they happen. When individuals have a history of engaging in an activity (behavior) and are injured (punished), they may avoid similar activities (behaviors) to limit the possibility (negative reinforcement) of reinjury. It is important to explore with the individual what need they are trying to meet by being inactive. High fears of reinjury invoke high feelings of anxiety and worry that activity will make things worse.

- Why are you afraid of hurting yourself?
- Have you reinjured yourself before?
- Has something a doctor said scared you?
- What messages are your body and mind sending you about your pain?
- Is your fear/avoidance helping you right now?
- Do your fears keep you safe or lead to being stuck, or both?
- Are you afraid your pain will get worse?
- Are you afraid your pain will not settle down or will take a long time to do so?

Negative feedback loop

Chronic pain can change an individual's thoughts, feelings, and actions. Pain can lead to a series of experiences that actually make the original pain worse. An example of what this cycle is and how it works may be helpful. A young man is experiencing chronic back pain caused from a work injury (initial event). He cannot do many of the things that he used to do in the same way and becomes frustrated (response). He focuses on all the things he has lost and feels demoralized (loss of hope). He believes that his future involves living the exact same way he is now (demoralization). He is miserable and tells himself that nothing will ever change (negative self-talk). When he has opportunities to engage in things he likes to do, he states he does not want to get hurt or take a chance to do so (avoidance). He sits by himself and wishes things were different (inactivity and isolation). Things change very little for him (reality). Since there is very little change he worries that things could get worse if he did something different, so he avoids activities that could cause him pain (negative reinforcement) out of fears of reinjury. The constant fear and avoidance leads to worry and further inactivity (loss of motivation). He starts to question whether his treatment is working and does not follow his team's suggestions (lack of compliance). Things continue to get worse and he questions why. This is an extreme example, but many individuals can relate to multiple parts of this cycle in either urge or action.

Teaching skills (T)

The suggested skills to teach in this session are designed to assist the individual in recognizing their pain triggers and to create a plan to cope more effectively. It is suggested to use the **Skills Implementation Plan (SIP)** for this exercise to create a proactive plan. The form can be used to identify either a situation from the past or one similar that the individual anticipates happening in the future. An action plan can then be created to guide the individual's attempts to cope with situations more effectively.

Observe – Noticing one's experience
Describe – The process of putting words on one's experience
Participate – Noting what the individual is doing to cope with the current situation and how present they are in the process

When these skills are used in combination or in a linear fashion, they provide a process to recognize patterns of thoughts and behaviors. They can be used to identify how an individual interprets, reacts, and attempts to cope with an event. This promotes increased awareness and pattern recognition skills to be able to identify pain triggers from past situations and thereby better anticipate them happening again in the future. Once this has been completed, they can apply the skill of **Effectively**.

Effectively – Needs are being met in a safe and healthy manner

This skill is important to teach and review when identifying whether the individual's current functioning is optimal or acceptable. Observe, describe, and participate provides information about patterns and where the individual is in the stages of change process. Effectively provides information about how effective the individual is being. If what they are doing meets their needs in a safe and healthy manner, continue the plan. If what they are currently doing does not meet these criteria, review and potentially modify the **SIP Form**.

For some individuals, it may be more effective for them to review situations that have already happened. This allows for learning from past experience to create a proactive coping plan.

Many individuals struggle with modifying activities. A key point of discussion is to review frequency (F) of the activity, intensity (I) of engagement, and duration (D) of involvement. Introduce the concept of altering aspects of FID through attempts at self-regulation and pacing strategies.

"Fight" is a common coping response that may be defined as: continuing to participate in an activity until its completion regardless of the pain that is experienced or produced. Many individuals tend to cope with events by "powering-through." They tend to disregard their pain triggers and continue with the activity.

"Flight" is a common coping response that may be defined as disengaging from an activity that begins to trigger a pain response. This may be very healthy at times, but may also lead to stopping an activity out of fear that a pain response may happen. This concept also includes disengaging from an activity in the anticipation that pain may be triggered.

"Freeze" is a common coping response that may be defined as avoiding any activity that may lead to a pain response. Many individuals choose to avoid activities that have no history of causing pain out of fear that pain may occur, so it is safer to avoid the entire situation.

It is important to introduce a "Behavior Chain" to assist the individual in identifying their responses to activities that may or may not affect their pain levels. This allows for review of the antecedents, the response of the individual, and the generation of behavioral alternatives that target increases in adaptive functioning.

Applying skills and concepts (A)

- Introduce/discuss the homework assignment on **Turning Fear and Inactivity Into Action and Hope**
- Review homework from previous session
- Problem-solve barriers to this process

Generalizing skills and concepts (G)

- Problem-solve barriers to creating an action plan for **Turning Fear and Inactivity Into Action and Hope**
- Assign homework on the individual's action plan (**Turning Fear and Inactivity into Action and Hope, Behavior Chain, SIP Form**)

Notes to clinicians and individuals

- It is important to review the differences between reinjury and soreness from healthy engagement in activities.
- Action is a key to health. Movement and activity are important to physical and mental health.
- History is a guide *for* the future; it is not an exact predictor *of* it.
- Fears can serve as motivation for change, avoidance, and stagnation.
- Trading fear for pain is not a fair trade.
- Fear is a powerful emotion commonly associated with pain.
- Negative cycling affects us all; limiting its impact is a key clinical target.
- Start with validation to avoid defensiveness.

Social Curriculum

Session focus: Managing conflict

TAG
Teach – Apply – Generalize

- The goal of this session is to
    - Have individual's learn how to manage conflict more effectively
    - Increase effective skill use in relationships
- What to discuss:
    - Conflict resolution
    - Positive consequences of conflict
    - Negative consequences of conflict
- Skills to teach
    - Dear Man
    - Give
    - Fast
    - MAD
- Generalize
    - Create an action plan for **Managing Conflict**
    - Problem-solve
    - Commit to their plan
    - Review in next session
- Review goal sheet

Managing conflict

Introduction of the topic
Learning how to manage conflict in a healthy manner is very difficult for many individuals. Conflict is inevitable; it is not *if* it is going to happen, but a question of *when* it will happen. Individuals argue about many different things ranging from personality differences to disputes over daily tasks. When individuals are in pain or distress, their frustration tolerance is lowered and many things can be a focal point for disagreements. "Small" things and "major" life events can trigger disagreements. It is important to be able to disagree in a healthy manner or manage conflict when it occurs without damaging relationships. Conflict is common in relationships and serves many functions, both positive and negative.

Positive consequences of conflict
Not all conflict is "bad." There are many positives that can come from conflict in a relationship if it is managed effectively. Without conflict, relationships would be stagnant and there would be no growth for the relationship itself. When individuals are being open and honest (which builds trust) in relationships, they are able to

explore how to have differences in a safe way. They are able to practice accepting others for who they are. They have opportunities to learn from others who think and behave differently than them. Individuals are exposed to new ideas and experiences by being with others who are different. There are opportunities to have disagreements and practice building and repairing relationships. There are times that relationships need to be ended for the health of the individuals who are involved. This allows for exposure to guilt, grief, distress, and loss. When individuals are able to manage the emotions and demands of relationships their lives tend to be happier and more fulfilling.

Negative consequences of conflict

There are also many negatives that come from conflict in relationships if that conflict is not managed effectively. Individuals can become very emotional and act from a place of anger. This may break the trust in relationships and can become aggressive. Conflict can be used to control or intimidate others. Individuals are exposed to intense and painful emotions. This can lead to impulsive behaviors and hurtful comments. Conflict can also be habitual and slowly erode the value of the relationship, causing it to end. People leave, which can trigger anxiety, fear, guilt/shame, and loss. Individuals can feel unsupported and invalidated. It is common to withdraw out of fear that conflict will happen. Avoiding situations can lead to being distant and emotionally unavailable. Conflict in relationships can lead to neglecting others and the relationship itself. It can also make physical and psychological pain worse.

Teaching skills (T)

The suggested skills to teach in this session are designed to assist the individual to manage conflict in relationships more effectively.

The first sets of skills to teach are **Dear Man (DM)**, **Give (G)**, and **Fast (F)**. These skill sets are designed to work toward healthier relationships. They are most effective when used in combinations with each other. If asking for something or setting limits and boundaries, **DM** is a prioritized skill with **G** and **F** being used as supportive or ancillary skills. If the situation requires the individual to build or maintain a relationship, **G** would be the prioritized skill with **DM** and **F** being used as supportive or ancillary skills. If the situation requires the individual to focus on their self-esteem or self-concept, **F** is a prioritized skill with **DM** and **G** being used as supportive or ancillary skills.

Assertiveness training is a key component to setting limits and boundaries or asking for something the individual wants. The skill set of **DEAR MAN (DM)** is designed to teach the individual to increase the probability of getting their wants or needs met.

Describe – Use Observe and Describe to summarize the situation and identify the facts that support the request or reason for setting a limit or boundary.
Express – Share your beliefs or opinions when relevant or required.
Assert – Ask clearly for what you want or need.
Reward – Let others know how helping you meet your wants or needs will potentially impact their situation.

Mindful – Stay focused on your request and avoid leaving the topic.

Act confident – Use an assertive tone, have confident body language, make eye contact, and stay calm.

Negotiate – Be willing to compromise to meet your wants or needs.

To apply the skill set of DM, the individual needs to first prioritize their needs. Make sure that the person you are communicating with has the capability of providing for the request. Take into account if the individual will respect the limit or boundary that is being established. Be aware of asking the right person at the right time. Consider if it is appropriate to ask for something given the status of the current relationship. It is also important to review whether the request meets short-term wants/needs or long-term wants/needs. This is an important set of skills to apply when needing to manage conflict in relationships.

The skill set of **GIVE (G)** is designed to teach the individual to build and maintain relationships.

Gentle – Be respectful in your approach and avoid threats, demands, and attacks.

Interested – Listen to the other person and be open to the information they have to provide.

Validate – Acknowledge and attempt to understand the other person's perspective.

Easy Manner – Be political and treat others in a kind and relaxed manner.

This is an important skill set to apply in addressing an individual's relationships with him/herself and others. The focus of this skill is to have the individual validate his or her own experience. When this skill is applied effectively, it decreases the need to rely on others for validation that they may not provide. The skill can assist individuals in reducing the impact of conflict in their relationships.

The skill set of **FAST (F)** is designed to teach the individual how to have self-respect and self-worth. This can promote a healthier and more positive self-image. As a result, the individual may be less vulnerable to compromising their values and taking a passive role in relationships.

Fair – Be fair to yourself and others.

Apologies – Do not engage in unnecessary apologetic behavior.

Stick to values – Use your own value system as a guide for your behavior.

Truthful – Be honest and accountable to yourself and others.

The skill set of **MAD (M)** is designed to manage conflict as it occurs. This skill set is similar to taking a time-out and interrupts the process of intense conflict.

Minimize – Acknowledge that conflict is occurring and minimize the chances of acting from a state of anger. Go to a different room or location, let the other person know when you will return to continue working on the issue, and find ways to "cool off."

Assess – Identify the level of your emotional distress and the intensity of the engagement. Prioritize the skills of DM, G, and F. Create a plan to re-engage when you and the other person are *both* ready to continue. If the situation is still intense, repeat the first skill until a safe and productive conversation can occur.

Damage control – Do not engage in hurtful words or actions. Do not allow yourself to be hurt or treated in a disrespectful manner. Repeat the two previous skills as needed.

Applying skills and concepts (A)

- Introduce/discuss the homework assignment on **Managing Conflict**
- Review homework from previous session
- Problem-solve barriers to this process

Generalizing skills and concepts (G)

- Problem-solve barriers to creating an action plan for **Managing Conflict**
- Assign homework on the individual's action plan

Notes to clinicians and individuals

- Time-outs aren't just for children – use your **MAD** skills.
- Have individuals share their experiences with conflict when they have experienced both positive and negative consequences.
- Many individuals use skills when experiencing conflict, but they may struggle to prioritize which skill will be most effective – PRACTICE – PRACTICE – PRACTICE.
- Assist individuals to identify what triggers conflict and how they immediately respond. This can help to identify where skills can be applied most effectively.

Session focus: The 3 Is: Identity/Isolation/Insecurity

TAG
Teach – Apply – Generalize

- The goal of this session is to
  - Increase the individual's functioning in relationships
  - Learn coping skills to improve the individual's functioning in the areas of coping effectively with themselves and others
- What to discuss:
  - How each of the 3 Is impact relationships
  - Identity
  - Insecurity
  - Isolation
- Skills to teach
  - Fast
  - Wise Mind
  - Opposite to Emotion – Action
- Generalize
  - Create an action plan to address one of the **3 Is**
  - Problem-solve
  - Commit to their plan
  - Review in next session
- Review goal sheet

The 3 Is

Introduction of the topic

Identity Identity may be defined as the unique features or personality of an individual. This means that all individuals are unique and have distinct differences from other people. Issues with chronic pain and mental health can challenge an individual's identity. They become labeled as a "patient" or "consumer." They are referred to by their injury or illness. It is also common to be labeled by the procedures they have done – an individual might be labeled "a total knee" or just "client." Labels serve a function of conveying a lot of information quickly. This is typical when individuals are working with insurance companies and professionals. Labels also present challenges. It may make the individual feel as if they *are* their illness. They may feel as if they are being talked *at* and *about* instead of being talked *to*. Labels also dehumanize individuals. Individuals can feel disconnected from their teams and supports. Many individuals may feel as if things are happening *to* them instead of making decisions *with* others. These examples can all challenge an individual's sense of identity.

Insecurity When individuals are struggling with the many challenges presented by chronic pain and mental health, it is common to respond by reaching out for support. There are many new experiences that are unfamiliar and threatening. Feeling insecure is a natural response when feeling threatened, unsure, and afraid. Many individuals access their support systems of professionals and personal supports such as family, friends, and groups of people faced with similar challenges. This can become problematic when their requests for support are too taxing on the current support systems that they have access to. There may be many phone calls placed to professionals in an attempt to get some of their questions answered. Professionals tend to be busy and may not be able to return calls in a timely manner. When contact is made, the calls may be rushed or there may not be "good" or acceptable answers to all of the questions. Repeated attempts may lead to labels such as "problematic patient" or "difficult client." This situation can make fears worse. Personal support systems can also be threatened. Individuals may become too "needy" or "clingy" when seeking support or reassurance. Individuals may feel guilt and shame as a result and respond by intensifying their attempts to gain support, or they may withdraw and feel rejected and unloved.

Isolation   Feelings of fear, insecurity, and rejection commonly lead to urges for isolation. When individuals do not feel understood, supported, or connected, they tend to withdraw from others into isolation. It is important to separate urges from action. Individuals may have the urge to isolate, but the state of isolation is attained through the action of withdrawing. Isolation is a protective state of being for many individuals. It may feel safer to be in isolation than around others. This can become problematic when the act of withdrawing is reinforced and becomes habit. If an individual feels threatened in some way, has an urge to isolate, acts on the urge, and feels safer by avoiding the threatening situation, they are more apt to repeat this process. Being in the state of isolation may feel safer for a short period of time, but as with other avoidance strategies, there are many negatives attached to this coping strategy. Being in the state of isolation can lead to catastrophizing, rumination on fears, becoming disconnected from others, not accessing needed supports and services, and worsening other symptoms of depression and anxiety. The state of isolation can be viewed as practicing the symptoms of pain and distress.

Teaching skills (T)

The suggested skills to teach in this session are designed to assist the individual in coping more effectively with identity, insecurity, and isolation.

The first skill set to teach in this session may be applied to working with the individual's identity. The skill set of **FAST (F)** is designed to teach the individual how to have self-respect and self-worth. This can promote a healthier and more positive self-image. As a result, the individual may be less vulnerable to threats to their identity.

Fair – Be fair to yourself and others.
Apologies – Do not engage in unnecessary apologetic behavior.
Stick to values – Use your own value system as a guide for your behavior.
Truthful – Be honest and accountable to yourself and others.

It is important to have individuals act through their existing roles to challenge the impact of labeling. Act as a mother/father, son/daughter, and challenge labels when they are experienced. Identify the current values that are relevant to the situation and use language and actions that represent those values. This humanizes the situation and provides challenges to labeling and stigma. If an individual behaves like an individual they increase the probability that others will treat them accordingly.

The concept of **Wise Mind (WM)** can be used to find balance between feelings of security and insecurity.

The concept of **WM** represents a balance between emotion and reason. Individuals experience three primary states of mind that all have different strengths and vulnerabilities: emotion mind, reason mind, and Wise Mind. It is easier to explain these concepts when they are placed on a continuum.

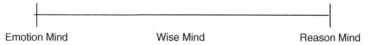

| Emotion Mind | Wise Mind | Reason Mind |

Emotion Mind – The state of mind where emotions are the primary influence on thoughts and behaviors. It represents a state of imbalance where individuals may be very creative, but also highly impulsive and reactive. When individuals are feeling insecure, they are emotionally reactive and not thinking clearly.

Reason Mind – The state of mind where the individual is logical, thinking, and rational. It represents a state of imbalance where individuals can be "cool, planful, and calculating," but they are quite distanced from their emotions and may not be aware of how their emotions are influencing them. When individuals are feeling insecure, moving into reason mind may provide initial distance from painful emotions, but may lead to catastrophizing and rumination.

Wise Mind – The state of mind where emotions and thoughts are balanced. It represents a healthy combination of thinking and feeling which is a goal-state for therapy. When individuals are feeling insecure, finding balance allows them to validate their own experience and select behaviors with a higher probability of meeting their needs in an effective manner.

The second set of skills is designed to assist the individual to cope more effectively with urges to isolate. The goal is to be able to identify the urge to isolate, and replace the behavior of withdrawing with behaviors that promote connection with others.

Opposite to Emotion (O2E) – Use opposite actions to avoid negative emotions. If the individual experiences the urge to isolate, they can engage in activities that connect them to others. They are acting opposite to their urge to isolate and that will not only change their behaviors, but will typically change the outcome and not lead to isolation. Have individuals create a list of possible actions that assist them to connect with their support systems. Applying the skill of **O2E** interrupts the isolation cycle and replaces the withdrawal behaviors with healthier actions.

Applying skills and concepts (A)

- Introduce/discuss the homework assignment on **The 3 Is**
- Review homework from previous session
- Problem-solve barriers to this process

Generalizing skills and concepts (G)

- Problem-solve barriers to creating an action plan for **The 3 Is**
- Assign homework on the individual's action plan

Notes to clinicians and individuals

- It is expected that many individuals will struggle with all three of the issues presented in this session. Prioritize the needs and address them in order.
- Multiple skill sets are relevant to the work in this session. Have individuals consult the **Master Skills Sheet** to assist in customizing the interventions.
- Changing behaviors is a key to the work in this session. It is important to interrupt the negative cycles in thought and behavior as a first step for possible interventions. Then healthier thoughts and behaviors can be introduced to replace ineffective ones.
- Validate the impact of the 3 Is before working toward change.
- Finding balance is quite difficult, but can be accomplished through consistent skill use and awareness.

Session focus: Problem-solving

TAG
Teach – Apply – Generalize

- The goal of this session is to
  - Increase the individual's problem-solving strategies and their effectiveness
  - Individuals will learn skills to cope more effectively in complex situations and with others
- What to discuss:
  - General problem-solving strategies
  - Watching others
  - Trial-and-error
  - One size fits all
- Skills to teach
  - Individual-based problem-solving model
  - Social-based problem-solving model
- Generalize
  - Create an action plan for **Problem-Solving Models**
  - Problem-solve
  - Commit to their plan
  - Review in next session
- Review goal sheet

Problem-solving

Introduction of the topic

Many individuals are never formally taught how to solve a problem. This can lead to increased frustration, mood reactivity, and social difficulties. When needs go unmet for an extended period, it is draining on the individual and their support system. This session is designed to assist the individual in learning effective methods of problem-solving. Most learning about how to solve problems typically happens in three different ways: by watching others, through trial-and-error, or by applying the "one size fits all" approach.

Watching others

Many individuals learn how to solve problems from watching others. Caregivers such as parents or family members teach certain methods to children on how to solve their problems. This is a very common and effective manner of learning. Others "model" certain approaches or behaviors. Typically, a specific process is taught. The learner watches the approach to the problem in a passive manner. There tends to be an explanation and discussion of the process, the anticipated outcome, and the value that may be influencing the decision. The individual then attempts to repeat this process when they are faced with some form of problem. One potential difficulty in this process is that the behaviors that are being modeled for the individual to learn may be quite unhealthy. The individual then repeats patterns of behavior that may solve problems, but may also hurt themselves or others in the process.

Consider an individual who wants to learn (problem) how to ride a bike (solution). The teacher in this scenario may tell the learner how a bike works, the importance of balancing and pedaling, and may demonstrate how a bike is ridden. The learner is then expected to practice what has been taught by following a specific set of instructions while visualizing how the end product (successful riding) was accomplished. The skill is then learned through practice and a few band-aids.

Trial-and-error

Many individuals learn how to solve problems through trial-and-error learning. This is where the individual is faced with a problem, and internally creates a plan designed to solve the problem. They act on the plan and evaluate the consequences. If the problem is not solved, they attempt to find an entirely new solution. Over time, and through multiple attempts at solutions, one eventually works and the problem is resolved. This can be a very effective method to apply to solving problems. Difficulties can and do occur with this approach, however. Trial-and-error leaning takes time to apply and may not involve input from others. Some problems require a quick and well-crafted plan. This style of learning does not consistently lend itself well to time-contingent and socially based problems.

Consider an individual who is having a problem going to sleep at night and as a result is very easily frustrated. Many different people and situations then trigger this frustration. A trial-and-error approach may target learning to interact with others differently. After reading multiple books on healthy relationships and anger-management, the individual finds more patience and acceptance with other people and situations. This has value in this case, but may not solve the underlying issue. As a result, the individual is more effective in their relationships, but is still not sleeping well, which was the initial issue that created the problem. Since the initial problem still exists, the individual will need to problem-solve additional strategies for other difficulties caused by a lack of sleep. This concept is referred to as "chasing fires."

One size fits all

Many individuals learn how to solve problems through a "one size fits all" approach. If an individual learns one strategy or approach to solving problems that works on the first try, it is common to try it again in a different situation. They have been reinforced by meeting a need or the removal of a problem. This can be a very effective way to solve problems. A problem happens when this one approach is applied to all situations or is done in a rigid manner.

Consider an individual who is arguing with a cashier at a store who did not allow them to return an item. When the individual became angry and started shouting, the cashier finally agreed to allow the return. The individual was reinforced for getting angry in a public setting. That same individual then yells at his or her children in the grocery store when they are holding their favorite cereal. They return the item, which is a reinforcer, but then the individual becomes uneasy when everyone is staring at them and their children are crying. Even though the desired behavior (returning the cereal) was accomplished, the end result (people staring and crying children) was not effective.

Teaching skills (T)

The suggested skills to teach in this session are designed to assist the individual to problem-solve in a more effective manner. Two different strategies will be taught to provide flexibility in both method and involvement of others in the process.

Individual-based problem-solving model
The first strategy is for the individual who is addressing a problem without the involvement of others. This is done in a series of steps, and some steps may need to be repeated and modified throughout the process.

1. Identify the problem
    a.   How is this impacting your thoughts, feelings and behaviors?
2. Review your values
    a.   Include your strengths and limitations
3. Determine all involved
    a.   This includes yourself, others, and your environment (systems you are involved with)
4. Brainstorm potential solutions
    a.   No possibility is thrown out
5. Consider the potential consequences of each decision
    a.   Narrow the possibilities and attach potential positive and negative consequences to each idea
    b.   Create a pros and cons list for each potential solution
6. Select and implement the desired course of action
    a.   Evaluate whether the plan is working and needs to be continued, or whether it is not working as planned and needs to be modified or stopped

Social-based problem-solving model
The second strategy is for the individual who is addressing a problem with the involvement of others. This is done in a series of steps, and some may need to be repeated and modified throughout the process.

1. Recognize the problem
    a.   What is the problem?
    b.   Why is it a problem?
    c.   Who is involved now and potentially in the future?
2. Define the problem
    a.   Create your own definition
    b.   Consider factors of age, race, gender, values, and power differentials
    c.   Get information and perspectives from others
3. Generate potential solutions
    a.   Brainstorm potential solutions
    b.   Create a pros and cons list for each potential solution

4. Select a potential solution
   a. Consider if the solution meets short-term, mid-term, or long-term needs
5. Review the process
   a. How did I reach this solution?
   b. Is the "golden rule" of "treat others as you would have them treat you" involved?
   c. Did I consider all of the relevant factors?
   d. What is my motivation for this decision?
6. Implement and evaluate the solution
   a. Is new information available?
   b. Do I need to continue, modify, or stop the plan?
7. Reflect on the process
   a. What was learned?
   b. How does this affect others, my environment, and me in the future?

Applying skills and concepts (A)

- Introduce/discuss the homework assignment on **Problem-Solving Models**
- Review homework from previous session
- Problem-solve barriers to this process

Generalizing skills and concepts (G)

- Problem-solve barriers to creating an action plan for **Problem-Solving Models**
- Assign homework on the individual's action plan

Notes to clinicians and individuals

- Have individuals complete both homework assignments for the same problem and discuss the reasons one model was selected over the other.
- It is important for individuals to be taught both models. There are times when one or the other will be more practical or effective.
- Both models address the barriers identified in the discussion section (healthy learning, timing, and generalizability).
- Focus on applying strengths to the anticipated barriers that individuals identify.
- Problem-solving is a skill that needs to be practiced in order to become proficient.
- Many skills can be used throughout both models; encourage creativity in skill use and application.
- Values and morals are key aspects of problem-solving. It may be helpful to have individuals complete an inventory on what their values and morals are.
- The reader is strongly encouraged to read Brody's (1993) work linking empiricism to scientific research and to review Hill & Harden's (1998) model on decision making, which is modified in this session.

Social Curriculum

Session focus: Nurturing support systems

TAG
Teach – Apply – Generalize

- The goal of this session is to
  - Learn coping skills to improve the individual's functioning in the area of nurturing support systems
- What to discuss:
  - Support systems
  - What is support?
  - Who is a part of my support system?
- Skills to teach
  - Building Positive Experience
  - Validation
- Generalize
  - Create an action plan for **Nurturing Support Systems**
  - Problem-solve barriers
  - Commit to their plan
  - Review in next session
- Review goal sheet

Nurturing support systems

Introduction of the topic
Very few individuals feel over-appreciated, over-valued, and over-compensated for their hard work and dedication. It is much easier to take positives in life for granted and focus our attention and efforts on what is going "wrong" in the moment. It is human nature to avoid pain and work toward minimizing distress. If most of an individual's time, effort, and energy is spent focusing on problems, support systems may feel neglected and taken for granted. This can be a recipe for disaster.

What is support?
Support is the act of bravely or quietly enduring something. It is staying with an individual when many others would leave. Support is providing assistance or help. It is engaging with another person and working with him or her toward a common goal, or completing a task. Support is promoting the interests or causes of another. It is working with another person on something they find important or valuable. Support is advocating and providing a firm foundation for another person. It is standing up for someone when they cannot do it for themselves. Support is providing motivation and guidance when someone stumbles or loses their way. Support is caring for another individual even when they find it difficult to care for themselves.

Who is a part of my support system?

There are many definitions of support systems and they are unique to each individual. Professionals can be part of a support system. Many professionals work to keep the individual's best interests and potential present in their interactions. Professionals perform procedures, provide treatment and information, and provide necessary objectivity and expertise in times of need. They provide care, compassion, and support.

Family members can also be part of a support system. Family members provide love, acceptance, and understanding. They assist with physical, psychological, and emotional needs. They are there when friends would have left. They perform tasks that no one else is capable of or willing to do. Family members advocate for individuals to help them with their rights and responsibilities. They share their experiences, hopes, and dreams. They share their fears and insecurities. Family members share their lives.

Friends can also be part of a support system. Friends provide many of the supports that are common to family members. Friends can assist in daily activities and provide a sense of connection. They can serve as advocates and confidants. Friends can also provide objectivity that family members may not be able to do since the relationships tend to be less emotionally involved. Friends are important parts of any support system.

Acquaintances can also be part of a support system. It may be easier to share information and experiences with people who are not involved in the individual's daily life. They may be able to connect on similar issues and provide a sense of normalcy and connection to "a bigger world." They may be part of a social group or members of a support/therapy group. They provide connection, shared interests, and diversity of experiences.

Barriers to nurturing support systems

There are many barriers to nurturing support systems. This list identifies many common examples and the potential hidden messages attached to each.

- I am too busy (You are not worth the effort).
- I never thought of it (I don't consider your needs; I am too focused on myself).
- They don't want anything from me (I am not worthy of them).
- We fight all the time (It is too much of a bother to do/passive-aggressive).
- Our relationship never needed this before (I want things to be like they were).
- I am in too much pain or distress to do this now (It's not worth the effort).
- I can't (I don't know how).
- I won't (I can do this by myself).
- I don't know how (It is easier to avoid than to learn).
- When do I do something for them (It's not convenient for me)?
- I don't have money to spend on them (I can only show caring by buying gifts).
- I just want to be left alone (Let me suffer).
- Things are just fine the way that they are now (Denying reality).

Teaching skills (T)

The suggested skills and concepts to teach in this session are designed to nurture an individual's relationships with members of their support system.

The first skill to teach is **Building Positive Experience (BPE)**.

Building Positive Experience (BPE) – Creating or engaging in activities that lead to positive moods. Invite others to engage in activities that are pleasurable. Holding hands, playing with children, going for walks. Find ways to spend enjoyable time with others.

This skill is designed to activate behaviors that serve two distinct purposes. It can activate behaviors that lead to positive emotions and nurture relationships, which is the primary goal. This promotes healthy activity and leads to more positive moods while building relationships. This skill can also be used to modify activities that have been avoided or stopped due to the impact of physical pain or psychological distress. The key is to have the individual modify their engagement in the activity instead of not participating in it at all. Modifying activities can also challenge the individual's patterns of all-or-nothing and black-and-white thinking.

A second skill set to teach is **Validation (V)**. Members of support systems often feel invalidated, neglected, and misunderstood. **Validation** is an effective skill to apply in working toward more connected and healthier relationships.

Validation – To acknowledge, confirm, authenticate, verify, or prove. This concept may be simple to understand, but is very difficult to apply in a consistent and effective manner in relationships.

What validation is: Validation is acknowledging others' thoughts, feelings, and experiences. There is no room for judgment, interpretation, rationale, or disbelief.

What validation is not: Validation is not telling others what they are thinking, feeling, or experiencing. It is not arguing with others, blaming them, or excusing what you are or are not doing.

A concept to teach or review is treating others with kindness. Find ways to acknowledge or thank others for what they do. Give others compliments randomly throughout the day. Notice the everyday activities of others and participate in them in some way. Acknowledge past efforts or attempts at support. Recognize the positives in others and take the time to let them know that they are appreciated. A little effort can go a long way!

Applying skills and concepts (A)

- Introduce/discuss the homework assignment on **Nurturing Support Systems**
- Review homework from previous session
- Problem-solve barriers to this process

Generalizing skills and concepts (G)

- Problem-solve barriers to creating an action plan for **Nurturing Support Systems**
- Assign homework on the individual's action plan

Notes to clinicians and individuals

- We all need support. This is difficult to acknowledge and accept, especially in times of pain and distress.
- "The devil is in the details" can be a nice reminder for individuals to recognize and acknowledge the everyday aspects of support.
- Encourage the individual to engage in random acts of kindness.
- Remind individuals of times when they may have felt unsupported and discuss ways to minimize the probability of the past repeating itself.
- Identify the positive aspects of feeling validated, understood, and connected to others.
- Remind individuals to act in a similar manner to how they wish they were being treated.
- Resentment and conflict do not provide permission to neglect those who care for us!
- Sometimes the best gift that can be given is time, attention, and caring.

Session focus: Social roles in relationships

TAG
Teach – Apply – Generalize

- The goal of this session is to
  - ○ Gain insight and information about the impact that pain and distress have in relation to the different social roles individuals have in their lives
  - ○ Learn coping skills to improve the individual's ability to cope effectively with establishing and modifying social roles
- What to discuss:
  - ○ Social roles
  - ○ Social role disputes
  - ○ Social role transitions
- Skills to teach
  - ○ Observe, Describe, Participate, Effectively
  - ○ Fast, Give, Dear Man
- Generalize
  - ○ Create an action plan to complete **Social Roles**
  - ○ Problem-solve barriers
  - ○ Commit to their plan
  - ○ Review in next session
- Review goal sheet

Social roles in relationships

Introduction of the topic
Relationships require a lot of time, effort, and energy to build and maintain. Depression, anxiety, anger, and chronic pain all provide challenges to new and existing relationships. Social role disputes and social role transitions are typically a part of the challenges faced by many individuals. A social role may be defined as a set of connected behaviors, rights, and duties that an individual experiences in a social situation. Social roles have permitted behaviors that are guided by what is socially acceptable. When individuals approve of a social role, they will make sacrifices to comply with what is acceptable, and will punish those who violate expectations. Anticipated rewards and punishment account for the reasons why individuals conform to role requirements. (Lemay 1999; Thomas & Wolfensberger 1999)

Social role disputes
Social role disputes may be defined as conflicts that occur when the individual and their support systems have different expectations about the relationship. These disputes can involve both internal and external conflict. The basic premise is that the individual is fulfilling a social role that has accepted behaviors, rights, and duties.

There is a certain status that is involved, and the individual has both positives and negatives associated with the role.

If an individual is a manager at a convenience store, they are engaging in a social role. Society has deemed this work as valuable in some manner. The individual has the status of being employed and has a position in the company as well as in society. Behaviors that are connected may include being respectful, showing up to work on time, and performing the tasks associated with the position. Rights may include access to a safe work environment, freedom from harassment or persecution, and being granted appropriate authority to perform the behaviors of the position. Duties may include the tasks unique to the role or position, and acting from a position of power and authority, and not abusing that authority. The individual is reinforced through being paid for their efforts (intrinsically – feels good to work, or extrinsically – financially compensated for that work). When others are not acting in an approved manner, the manager may need to correct or potentially punish the behavior to promote compliance to what is acceptable (giving an employee a written reminder that they are not to be late to work). In the example of a social role in a work setting, there is typically some degree of clarity provided to the individual in writing. There are policies and procedures to guide expected behaviors. There are performance evaluations to assist in the process over time. There are laws governing rights of employers and employees. There are job descriptions identifying duties and expectations. Most interpersonal relationships do not have such explicit rules and expectations. The roles are initially established through negotiation or some active process and may change over time. The individuals involved in the relationships may not agree to the initial roles or the changes over time. This lack of agreement may lead to emotional responses and conflict.

Social role transitions
Social role transitions may be defined as changes in acceptable behaviors, rights, and duties that occur when an individual's social role is altered. In the case of an individual who is coping with mental health issues and chronic pain, multiple role transitions may be experienced. The changes may not be anticipated due to changes in functioning, and may not be accepted or agreed upon by others involved. Many individuals do not know how to cope with the changes and this causes further emotional distress, increased amounts of conflict and loss of support, and role confusion. When an individual is functioning in the role of partner or spouse, there are certain behaviors, rights, and duties associated with the role. This may include shopping for groceries, having access to all of the personal finances, and managing the finances to be able to complete certain tasks. If there is a change in functioning stemming from mental health or physical pain, the individual may not be able to perform the accepted role. The role needs to be altered in some manner during this time of transition. This places stress on the individuals involved. Transition times can involve uncertainty, fears, resentments, and many other reactions. It is important to be able to identify the need for change, problem-solve potential solutions, and act on a plan to stabilize the situation and redefine the roles.

Teaching skills (T)

The suggested skills to teach in this session are designed to assist the individual in identifying their current social roles, address potential aspects needing change, and create an action plan to stabilize the situation and reduce emotional/relationship stress.

The first sets of skills to teach in this session are **Observe, Describe, Participate**, and **Effectively**.

Observe – Noticing one's experience
Describe – The process of putting words on one's experience
Participate – Noting what the individual is doing to cope with the current situation and how present they are in the process

When these skills are used in combination or in a linear fashion, they provide a process to recognize patterns of thoughts and behaviors. They can be used to identify how an individual interprets, reacts, and attempts to cope with an event. This promotes increased awareness and pattern recognition skills to be able to identify pain triggers from past situations and thereby to better anticipate them happening in the future. Once this has been completed, the individual can apply the skill of **Effectively**.

Effectively – Needs are being met is a safe and healthy manner

This skill is important to teach and review when identifying whether the individual's current functioning is optimal or acceptable. Observe, describe, and participate provides information about patterns and whether the social roles the individual is currently functioning in are healthy for them and for others. Effectively provides information about how effective the individual is being. If what they are doing meets their needs in a safe and healthy manner, continue the role. If what they are currently doing does not meet these criteria, review and potentially modify the social role, or the behaviors, rights, and duties of the role.

The second skill set to teach in this session is **FAST (F)**.

The skill set of **FAST (F)** is designed to teach the individual how to have self-respect and self-worth.

Fair – Be fair to yourself and others.
Apologies – Do not engage in unnecessary apologetic behavior.
Stick to values – Use your own value system as a guide for your behavior.
Truthful – Be honest and accountable to yourself and others.

When this skill is applied effectively, the individual can dismiss painful messages by relying on their own values and by treating themselves respectfully. It can also reconnect the individual to their own truth in their experiences. There is no need to apologize for what they are experiencing and know to be true for them.

The third skill set to teach in this session is **GIVE (G)**.

The skill set of **GIVE (G)** is designed to teach the individual to build and maintain relationships.

Gentle – Be respectful in your approach and avoid threats, demands, and attacks.

Interested – Listen to the other person and be open to the information they have to provide.

Validate – Acknowledge and attempt to understand the other person's perspective.

Easy Manner – Be political and treat others in a kind and relaxed manner.

This is an important skill set to apply in addressing an individual's relationships with him/herself and others. The focus of this skill is to have the individual validate his or her own experience. When this skill is applied effectively, it decreases the need to rely on others for validation that they may not provide. The skill can assist individuals in social roles with others that are being established, or are in the process of changing.

The fourth skill set to teach in this session is **DEAR MAN (DM)**.

Assertiveness training is a key component to setting limits and boundaries or asking for something the individual wants. The skill set of **DEAR MAN (DM)** is designed to teach the individual to increase the probability of getting their wants or needs met.

Describe – Use **Observe** and **Describe** to summarize the situation and identify the facts that support the request or reason for setting a limit or boundary.

Express – Share your beliefs or opinions when relevant or required.

Assert – Ask clearly for what you want or need.

Reward – Let others know how helping you meet your wants or needs will potentially impact their situation.

Mindful – Stay focused on your request and avoid leaving the topic.

Act confident – Use an assertive tone, have confident body language, make eye contact, and stay calm.

Negotiate – Be willing to compromise to meet your wants or needs.

To apply the skill set of **DM**, the individual must first prioritize their needs. Make sure that the person they are communicating with has the capability of providing for the request. Take into account if the individual will respect the limit or boundary that is being established. Be aware of asking the right person at the right time. Consider if it is appropriate to ask for something given the status of the current relationship. It is also important to review if the request meets short-term wants/needs or long-term wants/needs. This is an important set of skills to apply when needing to negotiate and establish initial or existing social roles.

Applying skills and concepts (A)

- Introduce/discuss the homework assignment on **Social Roles**
- Review homework from previous session
- Problem-solve barriers to this process

Generalizing skills and concepts (G)

- Problem-solve barriers to creating an action plan for **Social Roles**
- Assign homework on the individual's action plan

Social Curriculum

Notes to clinicians and individuals

- Individuals are in a constant state of change concerning their social roles.
- Role diffusion is common when individuals are in a process of responding to changes in functioning.
- It is important to prioritize the skills of **Dear Man**, **Give**, and **Fast** when creating or redefining roles. **Dear Man** can be used to set the boundaries of the roles, while **Give** can be used to promote health in the relationships, and **Fast** can be used to guide the individual in making decisions by following their values.
- Encourage individuals to identify other skill sets that can assist them in the process of addressing their functioning within social roles.
- The reader is highly encouraged to read Osburn's (2006) overview of SRV for further information.

Session focus: Intimacy

TAG
Teach – Apply – Generalize

- The goal of this session is to
  - ○ Gain insight and understanding into human needs/desires in relation to intimacy
  - ○ Learn coping skills to improve patient functioning in the areas of sexuality and intimacy
- What to discuss:
  - ○ Shifts in roles and responsibilities
  - ○ Added distress
  - ○ Communication barriers
  - ○ Changes in sexual feelings and contact
- Skills to teach
  - ○ Give
  - ○ **Intimacy in relationships**
  - ○ Individualized skills
- Generalize
  - ○ Complete the homework assignment on **Intimacy in Relationships**
  - ○ Problem-solve barriers
  - ○ Commit to their plan
  - ○ Review in next session
- Review goal sheet

Intimacy

Introduction of the topic

Intimacy may be defined as something of a personal or private nature. When many individuals think of intimacy, they think of sexual activity. Sexual activity may be personal and private in nature, but there is much more to defining intimacy than having a sexual relationship. Intimacy involves having trust in relationships. Creating close bonds with others that gives open and honest communication. The presence of shared interests, goals, and activities are also common to intimate relationships. There is also a high degree of respect and concern when intimacy is part of a relationship. Intimacy refers to both verbal and non-verbal ways in which individuals relate to one another and enjoy their unique sense of connection.

Issues with mental health and chronic pain can challenge intimacy in relationships in many ways.

Shifts in roles and responsibilities

Chronic conditions often bring about shifts in roles and responsibilities in families. Many of these changes are in response to a change in physical ability and/or a change in emotional availability. When an individual is no longer able to perform certain functions in their daily lives, intimacy can be threatened. People may respond by being angry, bitter, and resentful. They may perceive the relationship as being unbalanced and unfair. There may be a shift from partner or family member to caregiver. The individual may respond with feelings of guilt and shame which reduce the emotional connections between people. Finding balance is a key to adapting to change in a healthy manner.

Added distress

Coping with chronic conditions can add to the normal challenges of daily life. Unpredictable physical and psychological functioning can lead people to be guarded and wary. This can create an atmosphere of heightened stress. There may be many forms of stress present, including those associated with financial issues as well as less time available for pleasurable activities, and less available emotional energy. The additional stress also decreases the amount of mental energy that individuals have. It is important for individuals to learn how to manage their everyday stress to be present and available in their relationships.

Communication barriers

Psychological distress and chronic pain affect everyone in the family. Changes that are experienced may be permanent or short term in nature, but everyone feels the effects. Many of the changes may be uncomfortable to discuss. It is often easier and more convenient to avoid talking about issues that are difficult. Family members and support systems do not have all the information needed to be understanding, supportive, or challenging. The result is that people start making assumptions and healthy communication is interrupted or stopped. It is important for individuals to share their experiences with others in order to build and maintain intimacy in relationships.

Changes in sexual feelings and contact

Chronic conditions often affect sexual aspects of relationships. Side-effects of medication may cause a decrease in libido or sexual functioning. High levels of emotional distress may interfere with sexual desire or performance. Changes in physical functioning may cause changes in abilities and increase fears associated with flare-ups and relapses. Sexual contact is an important part of intimate relationships. Sexual contact does not need to stop if it was a meaningful part of the relationship before difficulties started. Individuals with chronic conditions can still experience pleasure from sexual contact in most instances. Working through such issues can actually bring partners closer together. When people face challenges together, they may experience a new sense of power, resolve, and closeness that is different to what they shared before.

Teaching skills (T)

The suggested teaching method in this session is designed to empower the individual to identify their challenges to intimacy and create an action plan to address them in an effective manner.

Have individuals review the homework assignment designed for this session. Have them brainstorm and create a list of skills that may be relevant to their issue(s). Each individual is to identify a skill that could be used to help him or her increase a sense of intimacy in a relationship of their choosing. The relationships may range from their doctors, to family members or support systems, and to partners. They are to begin working to complete the **Intimacy in Relationships** homework in this section, and present a part they are willing to share in the next section. They are then assigned their action plan as homework. This provides practice for discussing difficult topics and gives each individual a chance to teach a skill they find relevant to their unique situation.

One skill set that will be relevant and beneficial is **GIVE (G)**. This skill set can assist the individual in connecting with others in a healthy manner.

The skill set of **GIVE (G)** is designed to teach the individual to build and maintain relationships.

Gentle – Be respectful in your approach and avoid threats, demands, and attacks.
Interested – Listen to the other person and be open to the information they have to provide.
Validate – Acknowledge and attempt to understand the other person's perspective.
Easy Manner – Be political and treat others in a kind and relaxed manner.

Applying skills and concepts (A)

- Complete/discuss the in-session assignment on **Intimacy in Relationships**
- Review homework from previous session
- Problem-solve barriers to this process

Generalizing skills and concepts (G)

- Problem-solve barriers to creating an action plan for **Intimacy in Relationships**
- Assign homework on the individual's action plan

Notes to clinicians and individuals

- It is important for individuals to address one of the four barriers to intimacy. It is typical for individuals to struggle with more than one barrier. Start by prioritizing one barrier and then address others in the future, when time permits.
- Intimacy is not created overnight, but is a process that takes time and is built on trust.
- It may be important to discuss taking healthy and calculated risks. "Too much too soon" does not create a stable foundation and does not make up for lost times and opportunities.
- Stigma around sexuality may need to be addressed in the initial discussion section.

Session focus: Styles of Interacting

TAG
Teach – Apply – Generalize

- The goal of this session is to
  - ○ Identify how pain has impacted your styles of interacting with others
  - ○ Learn coping skills to improve the individual's functioning in the area of social interactions
- What to discuss:
  - ○ Definitions of interaction styles
  - ○ Needs and Barriers
- Skills to teach
  - ○ Active listening
  - ○ Applying effective skill sets (Role-Play)
  - ○ Introduce **Styles of Interacting**
- Generalize
  - ○ Assign homework on **Styles of Interacting**
  - ○ Problem-solve barriers
  - ○ Commit to their plan
  - ○ Review in next session
- Review goal sheets

Styles of interacting

Introduction of the topic
There are many different styles of social interaction. These styles are influenced by personality traits, situational factors, and what has been reinforced. Individuals develop styles of interacting over time. The styles have been learned through meeting some need, and have been reinforced. When an action meets a need and has been reinforced, the action has a high probability of being repeated. This session identifies some of the positives and potential problems with each style of interacting. The goal of the session is to identify when the style of interaction an individual is engaging in is not effective, and to create healthier alternatives.

Examples for discussion
In the list that follows an example is given for each of the many different styles of interaction. It is important to understand that there are many strengths inherent to each style. The examples are not based upon judgment, but observation of patterns of interaction that are designed to meet needs, but may be used in a rigid and inflexible manner. These styles may be very effective for the individual, but may not work well in social settings. It is common for individuals who experience chronic pain and mental health issues to be unaware of their patterns of interacting with others.

- **Personalizing** – An individual who over-identifies with the presented information and perceives that others are talking about them or that they are to blame for something.
  - ○ Need being met – The individual feels connected to others and involved in the interaction.
  - ○ Potential social barrier – Others may be annoyed by the individual making a situation be about themselves when that is not accurate. It can be a way to dominate conversations.
- **Fixing** – An individual who typically provides solutions to other people's problems even when solutions have not been requested.
  - ○ Need being met – The individual feels valued and productive by helping to fix a problem.
  - ○ Potential social barrier – Others may view the individual as being invalidating or superior because the solutions are unsolicited.
- **Cheerleading** – An individual who encourages others by being overly optimistic and attempts to provide motivation to others in an unwavering manner.
  - ○ Need being met – An individual feels supportive, helpful, and connected to others.
  - ○ Potential social barrier – Others may view the individual's attempts to connect as unhelpful, pushy, and overly optimistic.
- **Invalidating** – An individual who fails to connect to another person's experience and challenges or argues about what they "should" be experiencing.
  - ○ Need being met – An individual is attempting to clarify what is happening so they can connect with others.
  - ○ Potential social barrier – Others may feel hurt or misunderstood, causing them to disengage or withdraw.
- **Joining** – An individual who connects with other people through their pain or distress.
  - ○ Need being met – An individual is attempting to connect with others by sharing their experiences with a similar problem.
  - ○ Potential social barrier – Others may feel that the only topics for discussion center on pain and distress.
- **Tangential** – An individual who responds to others by connecting to minimally relevant aspects of the process or content of the interaction.
  - ○ Need being met – An individual is attempting to either connect with others, or change the topic of discussion.
  - ○ Potential social barrier – Others may perceive the individual as not following the conversation or as being uninterested.
- **Competition** – An individual who challenges others by competing with their stories and identifying with being better or worse than others in some aspect of their disclosures.
  - ○ Need being met – An individual can relate to aspects of the conversation and wants to relate their story to others' stories.
  - ○ Potential social barrier – Others may feel offended or devalued.
- **Masking** – An individual who hides or disguises their true experience and typically provides information that is not accurate to their own experience.

○ Need being met – An individual is attempting to appear competent and confident so they are not perceived as being vulnerable.
○ Potential social barrier – Others are not able to connect in a genuine manner.
- **Performing** – An individual who agrees with all feedback and challenges on a superficial level, and then either rejects change or attributes positives/blame to others.
  ○ Need being met – An individual is able to deflect the focus of attention and avoid real or meaningful change.
  ○ Potential social barrier – Others perceive the individual as being stubborn or resistant when "old behaviors or patterns" return once the pressure to conform is removed.
- **Externalizing** – An individual attributes credit for success or failure to others in a consistent manner.
  ○ Need being met – An individual is able to give others compliments or deflect responsibility and blame onto others.
  ○ Potential social barrier – Others may feel angry, blamed, or disrespected.
- **Help-rejecting complaining** – An individual identifies a problem and then dismisses all potential solutions.
  ○ Need being met – An individual is able to avoid changing or "being fixed" by others.
  ○ Potential social barrier – Others may perceive the individual as whining and not wanting the help and support that they are offering.
- **Finding extremes** – An individual uses extremes in language, thoughts, or behaviors.
  ○ Need being met – An individual is attempting to clarify and simplify their experience by deleting the complexity of the situation or experience.
  ○ Potential social barrier – Others cannot connect with a "middle ground" or common experience.

Teaching skills (T)

The teaching in this session is designed to be interactive through role-playing active listening skills. The suggested skills to teach are active listening skills. These skills can provide a foundation for healthy communication.

1. Pay attention. Be aware of your body language. Make eye contact and focus your attention on the other individual.
2. Be non-judgmental. Keep an open mind. Be open to new ideas and perspectives. Avoid criticizing and arguing.
3. Use reflective communication. Paraphrase key points that the other person is making. Reflect back to them what you have heard to promote understanding and interaction.
4. Ask questions. Avoid making assumptions. Get clarity and encourage them to expand on their ideas.
5. Summarize. Briefly restate main points and what you have understood them to say.

6. Reciprocate. Share your experiences and how you can relate to others. Keep it brief.

Applying skills and concepts (A)

- Introduce/discuss the homework assignment on **Styles of Interacting**
- Role-play active listening skills
- Review homework from previous session
- Problem-solve barriers to this process

Generalizing skills and concepts (G)

- Problem-solve barriers to creating an action plan for **Styles of Interacting**
- Assign homework on the individual's action plan

Notes to clinicians and individuals

- Styles of interaction are neither "good" nor "bad" and we all behave in certain ways. It is important to identify when the interaction styles are ineffective and find healthier alternatives.
- Individuals may need to consult those around them to assist in identifying patterns of interaction.
- Reducing the role of judgment can assist individuals to be open to feedback and willing to change.
- Finding a balance of what works for the individual and others is a goal of this session.

Chapter 4

Handouts and Homework

Goal Setting Handout

Vision of Recovery (VOR)

An individual's VOR is the first step in setting realistic goals. The VOR is the "bigger picture" for the individual. This is where the individual identifies what they would wish their lives to look like if they no longer needed consistent medical and mental health services at the level of intensity they are currently involved in.

This is where the individual has one of the first opportunities to identify their hopes and dreams. It provides an initial direction for therapy. It may also identify strengths and motivation to work toward positive change in their lives. Here are a few examples of questions the clinician can pose to the individual:

"What do you want your life to look like in the next few years?"
"What do you want out of life?"
"What do you want your life to look like when you are no longer in primary treatment?"
"Can you imagine what your life looks like when you are no longer in treatment?"
"What do you want your life to look like when pain or illness is no longer controlling your life?"

Goals

Once the VOR has been established it is time to begin working on defining the individual's goals. Goals may be viewed as the degree and direction in which an individual needs to work to move closer to their VOR. This is the first step in operationally defining an individual's treatment. Specific areas that reduce the individual's ability to cope more effectively or function at a higher level are identified for treatment. Timelines are typically attached to goals to establish review periods and

CBT for Chronic Pain and Psychological Well-Being: A Skills Training Manual Integrating DBT, ACT, Behavioral Activation and Motivational Interviewing, First Edition. Mark Carlson.
© 2014 John Wiley & Sons, Ltd. Published 2014 by John Wiley & Sons, Ltd.

thereby assess movement throughout the therapeutic process. This is the "middle ground" between the VOR and the specific steps to begin the process. It is important to incorporate the individual's own words to promote ownership in the process. If the clinician does not incorporate the individual in the creation process, this allows for externalization, decreased motivation, and less perceived control, all of which lead to demoralization and decreased hope. Perceived power and control are necessary ingredients for the promotion and reinforcement of motivation. Here are a few examples of questions the clinician can pose to the individual:

"What I need to work on to reach my VOR is . . ."

"My priorities for treatment are . . ."

"What I need to learn or do differently is . . ."

Goal Setting
BIO

Objectives

Once the goals have been established it is time to begin working on the specific steps that are needed to move toward the identified goals. Objectives are behaviorally written and measurable. Objectives tend to be most effective when they are stepwise and sequential. This step is typically where individuals identify their barriers to more effective functioning and are taught specific skills or coping strategies to apply in treatment and generalize to their lives. The timeframes for objectives are typically what the client will do each day or on a weekly basis. Progression may be to initially identify a pattern of functioning, identify strengths and barriers, teach the individual skills or coping strategies, have them apply them in the treatment setting, and assign homework for generalization with a tracking and review process. Homework and objectives need to be reviewed and worked on in each session to promote accountability and consistency. Here are a few examples of questions the clinician can pose to the individual:

"What I need to work on each day to reach my goals is . . ."

"The first step toward my goal is . . . followed by . . ."

"How will I monitor my attempts to apply what I have learned and track whether it was effective or not?"

Vision of Recovery

1. **Goal**
   a. Objective (step 1) _____

   b. Objective (step 2) _____

   c. Objective (step 3) _____

2. **Goal**
   a. Objective (step 1) _____

   b. Objective (step 2) _____

   c. Objective (step 3) _____

3. **Goal**
   a. Objective (step 1) _____

   b. Objective (step 2) _____

   c. Objective (step 3) _____

Goal Setting   NAME: _____
BIO

Goal Setting Homework

Step 1: Define:
My *goal* is to: _____

My *need* is to: _____

Step 2: Assets (what are the available resources you can use to achieve your goal):

_____

_____

Step 3: Barriers (what might get in the way of achieving your goal):

Barriers to my goal: _____   Skills I can use: _____

_____   _____

_____   _____

Step 4: Action Plan (what are your behaviors and their timelines to take action toward achieving your goal?):

Action Behavior: _____   Timeline: _____

Action Behavior: _____   Timeline: _____

Action Behavior: _____   Timeline: _____

Step 5: Report the outcome in session

What was the outcome? _____

_____

_____

_____

Goal Setting   NAME: _____
BIO

Skills Implementation Plan

Crisis Behavior:
List below behaviors, feelings, and situations typically associated with the crisis at each scale level.

0–1 **NO CRISIS**

List typical situation: _____

List typical thoughts, _____

Feelings,_____

Behaviors, _____

_____

_____

Skills to use: _____

_____

1–2 **EARLY WARNING SIGNS**

List typical situation: _____

List typical thoughts, _____

Feelings,_____

Behaviors, _____

_____

Skills to use: _____

_____

3–4 **SOME DISTRESS**

List typical situation: _____

List typical thoughts, _____

Feelings,_____

Behaviors, _____

_____

Skills to use: _____

_____

5–6 **INCREASED DISTRESS**

List typical situation: _____

List typical thoughts, _____

Feelings,_____

Behaviors, _____

_____

Skills to use: _____

_____

7–8 **INTENSE DISTRESS**

List typical situation: _____

List typical thoughts, _____

Feelings,_____

Behaviors, _____

_____

Skills to use: _____

_____

9–10 **CRISIS POINT**

List typical situation _____

List typical thoughts, _____

Feelings, _____

Behaviors, _____

_____

Skills to use: _____

_____

DIAGNOSES	SYMPTOMS

MEDICATIONS:

1. _____   Dosage _____

2. _____   Dosage _____

3. _____   Dosage _____

4. _____   Dosage _____

5. _____   Dosage _____

6. _____   Dosage _____

7. _____   Dosage _____

MEDICAL ALERTS _____

_____

CONTACTS: List people to call for support (List friends and Mental Health Team members to contact in the event of crisis)

Therapist: _____   Phone # _____

Psychiatrist: _____   Phone # _____

Case Manager: _____   Phone # _____

Friend: _____   Phone # _____

Other: _____   Phone # _____

Other: _____   Phone # _____

The Pain Scale.

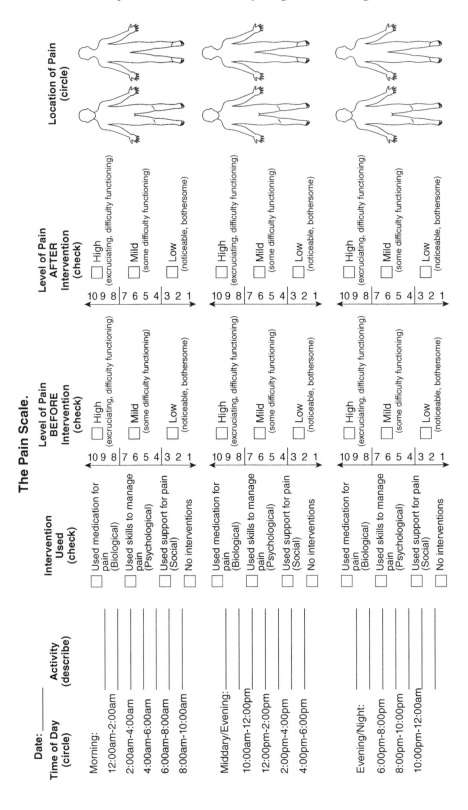

Sleep Hygiene   NAME: _____
BIO

Building a Routine Handout

There are several elements to building a healthy sleep routine. The individual is encouraged to practice these elements for at least one month in a consistent manner.

1. Go to bed when you are sleepy
   Do not force your sleep. It may be helpful to set a consistent time to start your bedtime ritual that assists in preparing you for sleep.
2. If you do not fall asleep after 20 minutes, you need to get out of bed
   Find a distraction that does not involve strenuous activity and is short in duration. When you become sleepy go back to bed. This may require a commitment to this process over and over until positive gains are achieved.
3. Get out of bed at the same time every morning
   You really want to minimize exceptions to this rule. Consistency is a stepping stone to healthy habits. The more we make exceptions, the harder and longer we have to work.
4. Establish a bedtime ritual that helps you prepare for sleep
   Engage in activities that calm the mind and body. Warm baths, scents, meditation, stretching, and reading are all effective examples. Notice that watching television is not on this list!
5. Keep your bedroom cool, quiet, and dark
   This promotes the 3 Cs of sleep – cool, calm, and centered.
6. Keep to your schedule
   Creating healthy habits takes time and consistency. Over time you will typically experience deeper, restorative sleep.
7. Avoid naps if at all possible
   If you must nap keep it to 10–15 minutes in length.

Sleep Hygiene　　　　　　　　　　　　　NAME: _____
BIO

Maintaining a Sleep Hygiene Routine Handout

1. Bed is for sleep so minimize other activities done in your bed
    Your bed is for sleep, not talking on the phone, watching TV, eating, or working on the computer.
2. Minimize or stop caffeine intake after mid-afternoon
    This will assist in keeping you calm and relaxed.
3. Avoid any alcohol consumption within 6 hours of bedtime
    Alcohol and deep, restorative sleep do not mix well
4. Avoid big meals or being too hungry before bedtime
    It is important to have balance with hunger around bedtime. If you need to eat, moderation is a key.
5. Avoid exercising 6 hours before bedtime
    Daily exercise is very important and needs to be done earlier in the day.
6. Have a plan to cope with worry thoughts
    Engage in deep breathing, visualization, or progressive muscle relaxation when agitated. Keep a notepad next to your bed to write your worry thoughts down and address them in the morning (practice letting go).
7. List strategies to get back to sleep
    Focus on relaxing your body and calming your mind. Engage in a quiet, non-stimulating activity.
8. Consult your doctor
    This is important to do before starting an exercise program and to assess if your sleep problems require primary medical interventions.

Sleep Hygiene   NAME: _____
BIO

Sleep Hygiene Homework

What steps do you need to take to improve your restorative sleep? Consult the Sleep
Hygiene Handouts to assist you with your plan.

1. Preparation: _____

    _____

    _____

    _____

2. If trouble occurs: _____

    _____

    _____

    _____

3. When to wake up: _____

    _____

    _____

    _____

4. Naps: _____

    _____

    _____

    _____

5. Maintenance: _____

    _____

    _____

    _____

Emergence and Patterns   NAME: _____
BIO

Baseline Assessment Form Handout

1. Establish a baseline of current pain through self-assessment.

    This is where the individual rates their pain on a 10-point scale with 10 being extreme pain and 0 being pain-free. The individual then selects a level of pain that is acceptable to them and at a level where they have effective coping strategies.

2. Review similar past activities by examining the frequency of engagement in the activity and how that affected pain levels.

    This is where the individual recalls similar situations and compares their current functioning to previous functioning when engaging in similar activities. The comparison between past and present may provide information on how frequently they engage in activities before their pain levels are pushed to coping threshold.

    If the probability for increased pain is high, the individual may need to decrease the frequency of engagement in the activity.

3. Review similar past activities by examining the intensity of engagement in the activity and how that affected pain levels.

    This is where the individual recalls similar situations and compares their current functioning to previous functioning when engaging in similar activities. The comparison between past and present may provide information on how intensely they engage in activities before their pain levels are pushed to coping threshold.

    If the probability for increased pain is high, the individual may need to modify the engagement in the activity through pacing or altering the activity itself.

4. Review similar past activities by examining the duration of engagement in the activity and how that affected pain levels.

    This is where the individual recalls similar situations and compares their current functioning to previous functioning when engaging in similar activities. The comparison between past and present may provide information on how long they can engage in activities before their pain levels are pushed to coping threshold.

    If the probability for increased pain is high, the individual may need to decrease the length of engagement in the activity. They may need to break down the task into smaller parts that can be accomplished over time in stages.

5. Analyze the data and attempt to predict the pain response given past experience and current functioning and ability.

   This is where the individual compares the present situation to what they have learned from the past. They create a probability for increased pain that is low, moderate, or high.

6. Complete a Pros and Cons list for engaging in the activity and for not engaging in the activity.

   This is where the individual decides if the "risk is worth the reward." They also review their current strengths and vulnerabilities.

7. Create/review their **SIP Form** or coping plan.

   This is where the individual creates or reviews a specific coping plan in relation to the activity.

8. Create the action plan and commit to its implementation.

   This is where the individual acts on their plan with no regret or remorse. They have done their best to analyze the situation and act accordingly.

Baseline Assessment Form Homework

1. Establish a baseline of current pain through self-assessment.

2. Review similar past activities by examining the frequency of engagement in the activity and how that affected pain levels.

3. Review similar past activities by examining the intensity of engagement in the activity and how that affected pain levels.

4. Review similar past activities by examining the duration of engagement in the activity and how that affected pain levels.

5. Analyze the data and attempt to predict the pain response given past experience and current functioning and ability.

6. Complete a Pros and Cons list for engaging in the activity and for not engaging in the activity.

	PROS +	**CONS −**
Engaging		
NOT Engaging		

7. Create/ review their **SIP Form** or coping plan.

8. Create the action plan and commit to its implementation.

Adherence to Treatment Protocols   NAME: _____
BIO

Self-Advocacy Homework (Medical Comprehensiveness)

Most of pain management is what *you* are willing to do rather than what your doctors can do for you. Remember, it is your pain, not your doctor's pain. You must be an individual and an active participant in your life, not just a "patient."

1. What could have been done for you to convince you that all medical interventions or treatments have been tried?

    _____

    _____

    _____

    _____

2. What do you feel could be done now to improve your medical interventions or treatments?

    _____

    _____

    _____

    _____

3. Do you have all of the medical information necessary to make your decisions?

    _____

    _____

    _____

    _____

4. What information might you need and where can you get the desired information?

    _____

    _____

    _____

    _____

5. What are your thoughts or beliefs about your current medications?

_____

_____

_____

_____

6. Are your current medications effective?

_____

_____

_____

_____

7. Are you experiencing side-effects that your doctors are aware of?

_____

_____

_____

_____

8. Do you believe that your medical team listens to you?

_____

_____

_____

_____

9. Does your medical team explain things in a way you can understand?

_____

_____

_____

_____

10. What are your current priorities that your medical providers need to be aware of and are they aware of them?

_____

_____

_____

_____

Complexity
BIO

NAME: _____

My Story – Part 1

Please share your story involving physical pain

What were you like before your pain started?

_____

_____

_____

_____

_____

_____

_____

What is your current relationship with your physical pain?

_____

_____

_____

_____

_____

_____

_____

MY STORY

Please share your story involving psychological distress

What were you like before your distress started?

_____

_____

_____

_____

_____

_____

What is your current relationship with your psychological distress?

_____

_____

_____

_____

_____

_____

_____

MY STORY

How does your physical pain affect your psychological well-being?

_____

_____

_____

_____

_____

_____

_____

How does your psychological distress affect your physical functioning?

_____

_____

_____

_____

_____

_____

_____

MY STORY

My Story – Part 2

(To be completed as a requirement for graduation from the program)
Please share your story involving physical pain

What was your physical pain like when you started this program?

_____

_____

_____

_____

_____

_____

_____

What is your current relationship with your physical pain?

_____

_____

_____

_____

_____

_____

_____

MY STORY

Please share your story involving psychological distress

What was your psychological distress like when you started this program?

_____

_____

_____

_____

_____

_____

_____

What is your current relationship with your psychological distress?

_____

_____

_____

_____

_____

_____

_____

_____

MY STORY

How does your physical pain and your psychological well-being currently affect your functioning?

_____

_____

_____

_____

_____

_____

_____

Please tell your story as you anticipate it happening for the next year.

_____

_____

_____

_____

_____

_____

_____

Functioning and Loss NAME: _____
BIO

Behavior Chain Analysis

Date:

What was the event? Who? What? When? Where?

_____

_____

_____

_____

What led up to the event? Give specifics of events, people, feelings, and beliefs.

_____

_____

_____

_____

What did you gain or expect to gain by making that choice?
(Emotional, financial, relationships?)

_____

_____

_____

_____

What were the benefits you gained by making your choice?

_____

_____

_____

_____

What were the negative consequences of your choice?
(for yourself, for others)

_____

_____

_____

_____

What skills could you use to intervene next time?
(What might you do differently? Think differently?)

_____

_____

_____

_____

Working With Your Team
BIO

NAME: _____

Keep It Real Handout

During the appointment, remember to **KEEP IT REAL**.

1. **K**ey in on the task at hand – You are attending an appointment with a professional. Be respectful and take an active role in your care.
2. **E**stablish the goals for the appointment – State your goals at the start of the appointment. It will be clear that you are taking an active role in your treatment and may help in structuring the appointment.
3. **E**stablish the available time – Ask the professional how long they *realistically* envision the appointment taking and pace yourself accordingly.
4. **P**rovide information – Present your tracking tools and the information you have gathered. This may also include your written list of questions. Be clear and specific.
5. **I** statements – Make consistent "I" statements and take responsibility for your decisions and care.
6. **T**ake notes – Write down the answers to your questions to help you remember them. You can also review them later.
7. **R**equest written materials – Gather as much information as you can. Information helps with making decisions and motivation.
8. **E**ngage in reflective communication – When a question is answered or you need clarity, let the professional know what you heard and check to make sure your interpretation and memory are accurate.
9. **A**sk questions – Be assertive. No question is too silly or stupid to ask. Do not leave the appointment with unanswered questions.
10. **L**eave with a clear care plan – Know what the next steps in your care are and discuss them with the professional before leaving.

Working With Your Team   NAME: _____
BIO

Keep It Real Homework

1. Prioritize needs and wants – Brainstorm needs and wants. Organize them
    into a list with priorities being at the top.

    #1 NEED: _____ #1 WANT: _____

    #2 NEED: _____ #2 WANT: _____

    #3 NEED: _____ #3 WANT: _____

2. Set clear goals and objectives for the appointment – Know the purpose of
    the meeting and specifically what you want to accomplish before the meeting
    ends.

    GOAL: _____

    What I want to accomplish today: _____

3. Create a list of questions for the professional – Organize your thoughts
    into a list of questions. Post them in an area that you frequently spend time
    in so you can add questions to the list as you think of them.

    Questions: _____ Answered? Y N

    _____ Answered? Y N

    _____ Answered? Y N

4. Organize the tracking forms and tracking cards – Gather the most recent
    and relevant information you have. This is one way to avoid seeming for-
    getful or vague.

    Do I have my Tracking Cards Ready?   Y N

    Do I have all of the most recent information ready?   Y N

5. Plan for childcare if needed – Ask a friend, family member, or the profes-
    sional's facility to assist. It is important to be able to focus your attention
    and be mindful during the appointment.

    Do I need someone to take care of my children?   Y N

    If Yes, who can I count on? _____

6. Plan or coordinate transportation – Make sure you have a reliable plan and mode of transportation. This is one of the first reasons individuals miss appointments.

   Do I need transportation for this appointment?   *Y N*

   If Yes, who can I call? _____

7. Plan for an advocate to attend if needed – Bring something to take notes on during the appointment. If this is difficult, ask if a friend or family member can attend to help you.

   Do I need someone there at the appointment with me?   *Y N*

   *If Yes, who can I count on?*_____

8. Visualize the appointment – Imagine yourself staying focused, active, and productive in the meeting. This will help increase your chances of getting your needs met.

   What will this appointment be like? _____

   _____

   _____

   _____

   _____

   _____

   _____

   _____

Working With Your Team   NAME: _____
BIO

Preparing for an Appointment Handout

Preparing for appointments is a very important activity. The individual can structure a set of tasks to complete before the day of the appointment.

1. Prioritize needs and wants – Brainstorm a sheet of needs and wants. Organize them into a list with priorities being at the top.
2. Set clear goals and objectives for the appointment – Know the purpose of the meeting and specifically what you want to accomplish before the meeting ends.
3. Create a list of questions for the professional – Organize your thoughts into a list of questions. Post them in an area that you frequently spend time in so you can add questions to the list as you think of them.
4. Organize the tracking forms and tracking cards – Gather the most recent and relevant information you have. This is one way to avoid being seeming or vague.
5. Plan for childcare if needed – Ask a friend, family member, or the professional's facility to assist. It is important to be able to focus your attention and be mindful during the appointment.
6. Plan or coordinate transportation – Make sure you have a reliable plan and mode of transportation. This is one of the first reasons individuals miss appointments.
7. Plan for an advocate to attend if needed – Bring something to take notes on during the appointment. If this is difficult, ask if a friend or family member can attend to help you.
8. Visualize the appointment – Imagine yourself staying focused, active, and productive in the meeting. This will help increase your chances of getting your needs met.

Structuring the day of the appointment can assist in this process as well.

1. Confirm childcare – Avoid last-minute chaos where possible.
2. Gather materials – Do not leave them at home.
3. Review the goals and objectives for the appointment – Remind yourself of the reasons for the appointment and what you want to accomplish.
4. Engage in a stress-management exercise – Take some time to relax and breathe before the appointment. Deep breathing, progressive muscle relaxation, and imagery can help to calm your nerves.
5. Leave at an appropriate time – Plan to be about 10–15 minutes early to your appointment. Being late can compromise your chances of having a productive appointment.

Orientation to Change   NAME: _____
PSY

Control vs Influence Homework

Control may be defined as having power over something (changing reality).

1. List 10 things you have control over

    1) _____

    2) _____

    3) _____

    4) _____

    5) _____

    6) _____

    7) _____

    8) _____

    9) _____

    10) _____

2. Which aspects of your physical pain can you control?

    _____

    _____

    _____

    _____

3. Which aspects of your psychological distress can you control?

    _____

    _____

    _____

    _____

4. How do your physical pain and psychological distress affect each other?

    _____

    _____

    _____

    _____

5. Which aspects of the combination of physical pain and psychological distress do you have control over?

    _____

    _____

    _____

    _____

Influence may be defined as producing some effect without exerting direct control or power (making things better or worse).

1. Create a list of 10 things you can influence.

    1) _____

    2) _____

    3) _____

    4) _____

    5) _____

    6) _____

    7) _____

    8) _____

    9) _____

    10) _____

2. Which aspects of your physical pain can you influence?

_____

_____

_____

_____

3. Which aspects of your psychological distress can you influence?

_____

_____

_____

_____

4. How do your physical pain and psychological distress affect each other?

_____

_____

_____

_____

5. Which aspects of the combination of physical pain and psychological distress do you have influence over?

_____

_____

_____

_____

Readiness to Change
PSY

NAME: _____

Readiness to Change Handout

The graph is designed to create categories for the individual to focus on. When distress is present, it may be difficult for the individual to understand the relationships they have between their pain and their functioning. This graph can provide insight and additional information to address in sessions. It can also show the complexity of relationships between pain and functioning while guiding the individual toward skill use.

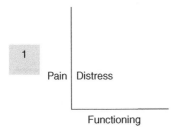

The X-axis is low to high levels of pain and the Y-axis is low to high functioning levels. When pain is present it causes distress, which in turn reduces functioning levels.

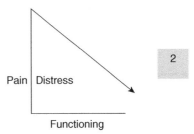

The goal is to decrease pain and increase functioning by reducing distress levels. The arrow indicates the goal of reducing pain and increasing functioning.

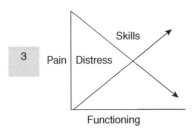

The mechanism of change is through the addition of skill use, which is represented by the arrow pointing upward. This indicates that functioning will increase when the individual becomes more effective with their skill use.

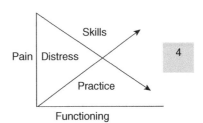

The key concept of practice is introduced to indicate that it takes time to practice new and existing skills to become more effective. Through consistent practice of the skills, distress will be reduced and functioning will be increased.

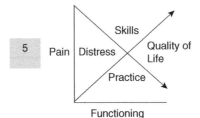

Quality of Life is now introduced. The more effective the individual's skill use becomes through practice, they will function at a higher level with less distress. The ending result is improved quality of life.

Depression
PSY

NAME: _____

Scheduling Positive Events Homework

	SELF	OTHERS
NIGHT		
EVENING		
AFTERNOON		
MORNING		

Pleased Homework

1. Describe your motivation to improve self-care skills (think of priorities, goals, and values)

    _____

    _____

    _____

2. Describe your strengths and resources to use PLEASED:

    _____

    _____

    _____

3. Describe your barriers to using PLEASED:

    _____

    _____

    _____

4. Describe the skills you will use to address those barriers:

    _____

    _____

    _____

5. Describe your action plan to start today (share your action plan with others and get started):

_____

_____

_____

6. Describe how your life would be different if you used effective PLEASED skills:

_____

_____

_____

7. Describe how you will acknowledge and celebrate your effective use of PLEASED:

_____

_____

_____

First Step Toward Change NAME: _____
PSY

First Step toward Change Homework

Just Noticeable Change (JNC) – Engaging in a behavior that leads to a change in focus or direction. This is a "baby-steps" skill. JNC allows for taking a first step toward change. It is a short-term skill designed to change the individual's "threshold" of experience. This helps the individual to identify that small steps can have a big impact concerning the process of change.

Provide an example for each of the following categories that you want to maintain or reinforce.

Thoughts

_____

_____

_____

_____

Feelings

_____

_____

_____

_____

Behaviors

_____

_____

_____

_____

Attitudes

_____

_____

_____

_____

Expectations

_____

_____

_____

_____

Beliefs

_____

_____

_____

_____

Anticipated outcomes

_____

_____

_____

_____

Provide an example in each category for which you want to take the first step toward change. Include that first step.

Thoughts

_____

_____

_____

_____

Feelings

_____

_____

_____

_____

Behaviors

_____

_____

_____

_____

Attitudes

_____

_____

_____

_____

Expectations

_____

_____

_____

_____

Beliefs

_____

_____

_____

_____

Anticipated outcomes

_____

_____

_____

_____

Anger Management   NAME: _____
PSY

Beliefs about Anger Homework

Validate each statement by finding an aspect that is true for you. Then challenge each statement by finding when the statement is untrue for you, or provide a skill to use to increase your effective coping strategies.

1. My anger controls me.

    a. Validation statement _____

    b. Challenge statement _____

2. I deserve better than this.

    a. Validation statement _____

    b. Challenge statement _____

3. I go from calm to angry in seconds.

    a. Validation statement _____

    b. Challenge statement _____

4. Anger is the same as aggression.

    a. Validation statement _____

    b. Challenge statement _____

5. I shouldn't be so angry.

    a. Validation statement _____

    b. Challenge statement _____

6. My anger scares me.

    a. Validation statement _____

    b. Challenge statement _____

7. My anger can't be predicted.

   a. Validation statement _____

   b. Challenge statement _____

8. My anger can't be controlled.

   a. Validation statement _____

   b. Challenge statement _____

9. My anger protects me.

   a. Validation statement _____

   b. Challenge statement _____

10. Nothing helps to calm me down.

    a. Validation statement _____

    b. Challenge statement _____

11. Other

    a. Validation statement _____

    b. Challenge statement _____

Managing Conflict   NAME: _____
SOC

Managing Conflict Homework

The skill set of **MAD (M)** is designed to manage conflict as it occurs. This skill set is similar to taking a time-out and interrupts the process of intense conflict.

Minimize – Acknowledge that conflict is occurring and minimize the chances of acting from a state of anger. Go to a different room or location, let the other person know when you will return to continue working on the issue, and find ways to "cool off."

Assess – Identify the level of your emotional distress and the intensity of the engagement. Prioritize the skills of DM, G, and F. Create a plan to re-engage when you and the other person are *both* ready to continue. If the situation is still intense, repeat the first skill until a safe and productive conversation can occur.

Damage control – Do not engage in hurtful words or actions. Do not allow yourself to be hurt or treated in a disrespectful manner. Repeat the two previous skills as needed.

1. What skills can you use to prepare for interactions that may lead to conflict?

    _____

    _____

    _____

    _____

2. How will you know when to use your **MAD** skills?

    _____

    _____

    _____

    _____

3. How will you know if your skills are effective?

_____

_____

_____

_____

4. Prepare your plan for potential conflict.

_____

_____

_____

_____

NAME: _____

Attributions Homework

Inaccuracies in attribution lead to misplaced blame and blind individuals to other potential causes. Aspects of your physical pain and/or psychological distress may be due to the following four distortions. Please provide an example of each where this is true for you and an example where this may affect your functioning in a negative manner (pain/distress generators).

1. **Covariation (relating)** – If a behavior or object is always present when another behavior or object is present they correlate, they do not cause each other to exist. An individual leaves their apartment or house at the same time each day to take a walk in the park. If a neighbor leaves at the exact same time each day to go to work, neither is causing the other to leave. They happen to have similar schedules.

   True: _____

   _____

   _____

   Pain or distress generating: _____

   _____

   _____

2. **Extremity (intensity)** – The more extreme the effect of a behavior, the more likely we are to make internal attributions. If an individual becomes angry and starts an argument that sends others running, they are more likely to consider themselves to be an angry person, not someone who is experiencing the emotion of anger.

   True: _____

   _____

   _____

Pain or distress generating: _____

_____

_____

_____

_____

3. **Discounting (dismissing)** – The more you know about environmental conditions surrounding a behavior, the less likely you are to make internal attributions. If an individual knows that their doctor is typically busy and has difficulty scheduling appointments, they are less likely to blame themselves when scheduling difficulties occur.

   True: _____

   _____

   _____

   Pain or distress generating: _____

   _____

   _____

   _____

   _____

4. **Augmentation (increasing)** – Motivation is increased if a barrier is experienced and overcome. If an individual fears holding their child, but does so even when there is a mild increase in pain, they are more prone to hold their child again even when fear is present.

   True: _____

   _____

   _____

Pain or distress generating: _____

_____

_____

_____

_____

Create a skills plan to reduce your vulnerability to one of these pain/distress generators.

_____

_____

_____

_____

_____

_____

_____

Meaning and Pain   NAME: _____
PSY

Finding Meaning and Purpose Homework

Physical pain

It may be viewed that individuals first relate to their physical environment which includes their awareness of their physical pain. When pain is present, it effects functioning. There may be limitations that are experienced, changes in abilities, financial problems, and increased risk of injury or illness.

Lack of meaning and purpose: _____

_____

_____

_____

_____

Meaning and purpose: _____

_____

_____

_____

_____

Social pain

Humans are social beings. Individuals relate to others in their world. This category of pain includes relationships, cultural issues, socio-economic issues, race identity, conflict with others, competition issues, and failure.

Lack of meaning and purpose: _____

_____

_____

_____

_____

Meaning and purpose: _____

_____

_____

_____

_____

Psychological pain

The psychological category includes how individuals relate to themselves and have their own personal sense of identity.

Lack of meaning and purpose: _____

_____

_____

_____

_____

Meaning and purpose: _____

_____

_____

_____

_____

Spiritual pain

This category includes the individual's attitude toward the unknown and how they assign meaning to experiences. This category also includes the individual's sense of connection to something larger than themselves. This is up to each individual to define.

Lack of meaning and purpose: _____

_____

_____

_____

_____

Meaning and purpose: _____

_____

_____

_____

_____

Guided Imagery Handout (Holtberg 2013)

The Guided-Imagery technique is a relaxation technique that allows you to refocus your attention away from your pain and symptoms and promote calming, relaxing sensations. These sensations can be very helpful in reducing the intensity of pain and have the added benefit of making you practice deep breathing and calm your own body to a more relaxed state.

There are several ways in which the Guided-Imagery technique can be used. Firstly, you can picture a place and imagine the details by yourself. You can also have a friend or family member read Guided-Imagery scripts or make a recording of a script and simply listen to it. Each way provides a different experience, promoting feelings of calmness and relaxation. You can learn new places to visualize, or even create your own images to allow a personalized experience of relaxation.

A scene for guided imagery

Take this time now to allow yourself to quiet your mind and focus on something other than the current moment. Allow yourself to be seated comfortably and begin to focus on your breaths. Notice the breaths you take as you begin to relax comfortably.

Begin to build an image in your mind now of a place where you are fully relaxed. This place is yours to experience and no one can bother you in this place. Imagine yourself standing in the grass on a steep hill. The grass is cool, prickly, and wet on your bare feet. As you stand at the top of this steep hill, you feel the warmth of the sun soaking through your shirt onto your back, toasting the skin on your neck. As you look down the hill you notice a small object, unclear of what it is.

As you proceed down the hill, you begin to walk slowly, feeling the prickle of the cool, wet grass beneath your feet. You begin by taking small steps, increasing your strides with the steep hill, feeling the pressure on your thighs and knees as you proceed slowly down the hill.

Once you approach the object, you notice it is a small, purple flower with yellow pollen. The flower has four small, almond-shaped petals. As you kneel down to be closer to the flower, you feel a cool, crisp breeze that blows your hair over your forehead. As you reach up to swipe the hair away, you notice the warmth of your fingertips touching your skin. As you look up, you notice more purple flowers, leading around a group of tall trees. As you begin to follow the path of the flowers, you notice a shadow behind the trees.

As you approach the end of the group of trees you feel the coolness of the shade the trees provide. With the sun now absent from view, you notice the hairs on your arm stand up in response to the coolness of the shade. Looking down you begin to smell the scent of the purple flowers, a light, sweet scent of floral. You begin to follow the trickling trail of purple flowers and notice once again the shaded object ahead.

As you approach the object you see that it is a brick wall, a rounded, tall, brick wall. As you walk closer to the brick wall you place your hand up against it, feeling the bumps, ridges, and cracks in the rough brick. As you pick up speed you can see the brick wall comes to an end. At the end of the brick wall you can see a tall iron gate. Once you reach the gate your hands grasp around the cool, hard iron, feeling the metal against your fingertips. Using your hands you push the gate open, hearing the creaking squeal of the gate opening.

As you proceed through the gate you notice a sound, a distant, bubbling sound of water. As you follow the sound you can begin to smell the water, the cool, musty smell of fresh water. As you move closer and closer to the water you can finally set eyes on a small, babbling creek. As you walk closer and closer to the creek you hear the noises of the bubbling water. Approaching the creek you bend down to take a drink, feeling the pressure of the rocks on your knees. Dipping your hand into the creek you feel the sharp, cold water against your hand and sweep the water up to your mouth. Taking a drink you feel the cold water traveling down your throat, quenching your thirst.

Now that you are refreshed, you begin back toward the iron gate, walking past the tall brick wall, through the trail of purple flowers and back up the hill, feeling your muscles worked, your thirst quenched, and your mind relaxed.

Take another deep breath and return to the moment when you are ready.

Tips for Guided Imagery

- If at any point you become uncomfortable, distracted, or discouraged, stop Guided Imagery and start at a time where you can dedicate a few moments to relaxation.
- Remember to breathe; count on your body's natural rhythm to keep you steady.
- Try various scenes to promote sensations from each of your 5 senses.

Progressive Muscle Relaxation Handout (Holtberg 2013)

This is one of the most widely used techniques that can assist in controlling symptoms. This process of tensing and relaxing muscles is easy and can be individualized to fit specific needs. One of the reasons muscle relaxation is so effective is that it produces immediate physical results that help us to recognize tension and release it, leading to better control of bodily pain. Another reason why muscle relaxation is effective is that it is easy to learn and easy to remember to practice across different settings. For example, muscle relaxation can be used at work, home, and can be done sitting or standing. Some of the sensations muscle relaxation promotes are increased relaxation, reduced muscle tension, increased calmness, and reduced overall pain.

There are many ways to practice muscle relaxation.

Start by sitting or standing in a comfortable position. Give yourself this time to focus upon your own body and allow yourself to experience recognizing tension and relaxation. The point of this exercise is to locate, identify, and experience tension and relaxation. Try to let all other noises and distractions go by. Close your eyes, this is YOUR time to focus on your body now.

First, begin by taking several deep breaths, comfortably filling your lungs and noticing your chest rise as it fills with air. Begin to notice your abdomen as they too fill with air. First your chest rises, and then your abdomen rise as you fill your body with air. Notice your breath, breathing slowly in . . . and out again. Take a moment to really notice your breath.

Now begin to focus your attention on your lower body. Notice your feet, the feet that carry your body. Notice the feeling in your feet. Begin to tense your feet now, curling your toes under, squeezing each muscle in your feet. HOLD this tension . . .

Now relax your feet. Notice the feeling between tension and relaxation. Next, notice the muscles in your lower legs, your calves, your shins, and your knees. Begin to tense your lower legs by tightening the muscles in your calves, shins, and knees. HOLD this tension . . .

Now relax your lower legs. Notice the feeling between tension and relaxation. Next, notice the muscles in your upper legs, your hamstrings and buttocks. Begin to tense your upper legs by tightening your hamstrings, thighs, and buttocks and squeeze these muscles. HOLD this tension . . .

Now relax your upper legs. Notice the difference between tension and relaxation in both of your legs from your thighs to your feet. Now notice your abdomen, the place in your body that houses your organs that give you life. Begin to tense your abdomen by squeezing your stomach muscles, your obliques, your sides and back, pulling yourself upward and tightening the core of your body. HOLD this tension . . .

Now release and relax. Notice the feeling between tension and relaxation, the difference between tension and relaxation. Now notice the muscles in your arms, your wrists, triceps and biceps. Begin to tense these muscles by squeezing only your arms and tightening the muscles in your arms. HOLD this tension . . .

Now relax your arms, noticing the difference between tension and relaxation. Now notice your hands. Your hands that are so useful to you. Begin to squeeze your hands together by making tight fists, using each finger, palm, and thumb of your hands tightening together. HOLD this tension . . .

Relax your hands, noticing the difference between tension and relaxation. Now, focus your attention on your neck, your neck that holds your head. Begin by tightening the muscles in your neck and squeezing those muscles. Squeeze your shoulder blades together and notice the tension. HOLD this tension . . .

Now relax your neck. Notice the feeling between tension and relaxation. Lastly, focus your attention on your face. Begin to tighten the muscles in your face, your cheeks, around your eyes, mouth, and forehead and tighten your face. HOLD this tension . . .

And now relax your face. Notice now the difference between the feelings of tension, the amount of energy your body uses to create the feeling of tension. Focus on the difference between the feeling of tension and the feeling of relaxation. Notice now your body completely relaxed. Your feet, legs, abdomen, arms, neck, and face, all relaxed. Allow yourself to enjoy the feeling of relaxation . . . Take another deep breath now, allowing your chest to rise as you take in air and slowly open your eyes and return back to the moment.

Some things to remember when practicing muscle relaxation:

- If pain becomes more intense, reduce the amount of tension you create.
- Let go of distractions, even if you hear noises or remember tasks uncompleted. Allow yourself these few moments to relax and focus on your own body.
- Once you feel comfortable with relaxing your entire body, then focus on the area of pain to relieve any painful areas effectively.
- Pick a quiet place and time during your day.
- Set realistic expectations for yourself and your relaxation, remember to practice.

Defense Mechanisms and Coping Styles Handout

- **Acting out** – The individual copes with stress by engaging in actions rather than reflections or feelings.
  - ○ Healthy – Feeling high levels of distress and turning energy toward walking, working out, or completing tasks.
  - ○ Unhealthy – Throwing temper tantrums, acting impulsively, being aggressive.
- **Affiliation** – Involves turning to other people for support.
  - ○ Healthy – Sharing your experience with others, asking for support or validation.
  - ○ Unhealthy – Having others do things for you that you can do, becoming dependent on others, losing independence.
- **Altruism** – Meeting internal needs through helping others.
  - ○ Healthy – Feeling high levels of distress and distracting yourself by helping a friend or neighbor, volunteering your time, becoming active in the community or with an organization.
  - ○ Unhealthy – Putting others needs before your own or engaging in self-neglect.
- **Avoidance** – Refusing to deal with or encounter unpleasant objects or situations.
  - ○ Healthy – Feeling high levels of distress and taking a break, distracting yourself for brief periods of time, doing something nice for yourself.
  - ○ Unhealthy – Sticking your head in the sand, pretending things don't exist, escaping, avoiding, or altering the distress.
- **Compensation** – Overachieving in one area to compensate for failures in another.
  - ○ Healthy – Feeling high levels of distress and turning energy toward things you do well, applying the **Building Mastery** skill, doing things to feel competent.
  - ○ Unhealthy – Masking, engaging in things you do well to falsely appear competent, pretending you are doing well when you are not.
- **Denial** – Refusal to acknowledge or recognize reality. Individuals who abuse drugs or alcohol often deny that they have a problem, while victims of traumatic events may deny that the event ever occurred.
  - ○ Healthy – Feeling high levels of distress and applying the skill **Push Away**, leaving a situation for a short period of time with a plan to return and address the distress.
  - ○ Unhealthy – Leaving a situation with no plan to return or address distress, denying what is real and letting your problems build, invalidating your own experience.
- **Devaluation** – Dealing with distress by attributing exaggerated negative qualities to yourself or others.

- ○ Healthy – Feeling high levels of distress and applying the **Comparisons** skill to *aspects* or *objects* that are involved in order to be able to take small steps to address the situation or distress.
- ○ Unhealthy – Decreasing your self-esteem, hurting others, or minimizing the impact of the distress.
- **Displacement** – Taking out frustrations, feelings, and impulses on people or objects that are less powerful or less threatening.
  - ○ Healthy – Feeling high levels of distress and punching a pillow, tearing a phone book, holding an ice cube in your hand.
  - ○ Unhealthy – Destroying property, "kicking the dog," making those around you feel miserable.
- **Projection** – Dealing with distressing emotions or situations by falsely attributing unacceptable feelings, impulses, or thoughts to others.
  - ○ Healthy – Feeling cool, calm, and calculating and identifying with the same qualities on others, treating others with respect when they are not being respectful toward you.
  - ○ Unhealthy – Denying your own experience by placing it on others, fearing someone will leave you and blaming them for being distant, feeling frustrated and accusing others of being angry.
- **Rationalization** – Explaining an unacceptable behavior or feeling in a rational or logical manner, avoiding the true reasons for the behavior.
  - ○ Healthy – Feeling high levels of distress and focusing on what you are doing well, engaging in positive self-talk, riding the wave of the current emotion and reminding yourself that the distress will not last forever.
  - ○ Unhealthy – Blaming others, attributing failure to the personal qualities of others, devaluing others when you feel hurt or rejected, or labeling your behavior as acceptable because others would act the same way.
- **Regression** – When confronted by stressful events, abandoning coping strategies and returning to patterns of behavior used earlier in development.
  - ○ Healthy – Feeling high levels of distress and simplifying your life for a short period of time, engaging in the skill of **Soothing through the Senses**, asking others for support and validation, having others take care of your needs for a short period of time to get a break from your distress.
  - ○ Unhealthy – Throwing temper tantrums, locking yourself in your room, becoming impulsive, acting out.

Defense Mechanisms   NAME: _____
PSY

Defense Mechanisms and Coping Styles Homework

Please provide an example of how you relate to each coping style. Attach one skill to each unhealthy example to improve your attempts to cope more effectively. Remember: these are common to most individuals. Challenge any judgment you may have.

Acting out – The individual copes with stress by engaging in actions rather than reflections or feelings.

Healthy _____

Unhealthy _____

Affiliation – Involves turning to other people for support.

Healthy _____

Unhealthy _____

Altruism – Meeting internal needs through helping others.

Healthy _____

Unhealthy _____

Avoidance – Refusing to deal with or encounter unpleasant objects or situations.

Healthy _____

Unhealthy _____

Compensation – Overachieving in one area to compensate for failures in another.

Healthy _____

Unhealthy _____

Denial – Refusing to acknowledge or recognize reality. Individuals who abuse drugs or alcohol often deny that they have a problem, while victims of traumatic events may deny that the event ever occurred.

Healthy _____

Unhealthy _____

Devaluation – Dealing with distress by attributing exaggerated negative qualities to yourself or others.

Healthy _____

Unhealthy _____

Displacement – Taking out frustrations, feelings, and impulses on people or objects that are less powerful or less threatening.

Healthy _____

Unhealthy _____

Projection – Dealing with distressing emotions or situations by falsely attributing unacceptable feelings, impulses, or thoughts to others.

Healthy _____

Unhealthy _____

Rationalization – Explaining an unacceptable behavior or feeling in a rational or logical manner, avoiding the true reasons for the behavior.

Healthy _____

Unhealthy _____

Regression – When confronted by stressful events, abandoning coping strategies and returning to patterns of behavior used earlier in development.

Healthy _____

Unhealthy _____

NAME: _____

Stigma Homework

1. Pain is a way to escape reality (avoidance)

    Validation statement _____

    Challenge statement _____

2. You are not tough enough (weakness)

    Validation statement _____

    Challenge statement _____

3. You are not motivated enough (resistant)

    Validation statement _____

    Challenge statement _____

4. You don't want to be fixed (broken)

    Validation statement _____

    Challenge statement _____

5. You should . . . (invalidating)

    Validation statement _____

    Challenge statement _____

6. You are living off the government (Freeloader)

    Validation statement _____

    Challenge statement _____

7. You're making yourself hurt so you can get drugs (addict)

    Validation statement _____

    Challenge statement _____

8. You are just a whiner (weakness)

    Validation statement _____

    Challenge statement _____

9. You are trying to avoid work (lazy)

    Validation statement _____

    Challenge statement _____

10. You are trying to get attention (needy)

    Validation statement _____

    Challenge statement _____

11. Your pain is not real – it's all in your head (faking)

    Validation statement _____

    Challenge statement _____

12. You're not really that badly off (catastrophizing)

    Validation statement _____

    Challenge statement _____

13. Your pain flares up at convenient times (manipulation)

    Validation statement _____

    Challenge statement _____

14. Other people are doing better than you are (minimizing)

    Validation statement _____

    Challenge statement _____

15. You are "crazy," "nuts," or "psycho" (devaluating)

    Validation statement _____

    Challenge statement _____

Chemical Abuse   NAME: _____
PSY

Living Life on Life's Terms Homework

There are many reasons why individuals abuse chemicals. When individuals discuss their chemical abuse, three main themes tend to emerge. These themes are the urge to escape, avoid, and alter their current reality.

Escape – feeling urges to escape the situation or one you anticipate to occur.
Avoid – feeling urges to avoid the situation or one you anticipate to occur.
Alter – feeling urges to alter your current experience, or one you anticipate to occur.

Identify five events or situations that trigger urges and circle your patterns of response.

1. _____

   Escape   **Avoid**   **Alter**

2. _____

   Escape   **Avoid**   **Alter**

3. _____

   Escape   **Avoid**   **Alter**

4. _____

   Escape   **Avoid**   **Alter**

5. _____

   Escape   **Avoid**   **Alter**

Identify one skill or intervention that may lead to a positive change in behavior in order to live life on life's terms more effectively.

Skill:
Application _____

Anticipated outcome _____

Skill:
Application _____

Anticipated outcome _____

Chemical Abuse Handout

Here are a few common questions individuals ask. The responses are from the Center for Disease Control and Prevention.

Why do some people react differently to alcohol than others?
Individual reactions to alcohol vary, and are influenced by many factors; such as:

- Age
- Gender
- Race or ethnicity
- Physical condition (weight, fitness level, etc.)
- Amount of food consumed before drinking
- How quickly the alcohol was consumed
- Use of drugs or prescription medicines
- Family history of alcohol problems

What health problems are associated with excessive alcohol use?
Excessive drinking, both in the form of heavy drinking or binge drinking, is associated with numerous health problems, including:

- Chronic diseases such as liver cirrhosis (damage to liver cells); pancreatitis (inflammation of the pancreas); various cancers, including liver, mouth, throat, larynx (the voice box), and esophagus; high blood pressure; and psychological disorders.
- Unintentional injuries, such as motor vehicle crashes, falls, drowning, burns and firearm injuries.
- Violence, such as child maltreatment, homicide, and suicide.
- Harm to a developing fetus if a woman drinks while pregnant, such as fetal alcohol spectrum disorders.
- Sudden infant death syndrome (SIDS).
- Alcohol abuse or dependence.

What is the difference between alcoholism and alcohol abuse?
Alcohol abuse[1] is a pattern of drinking that results in harm to one's health, interpersonal relationships, or ability to work. Manifestations of alcohol abuse include the following:

- Failure to fulfill major responsibilities at work, school, or home.
- Drinking in dangerous situations, such as drinking while driving or operating machinery.
- Legal problems related to alcohol, such as being arrested for drinking while driving or for physically hurting someone while drunk.
- Continued drinking despite ongoing relationship problems that are caused or worsened by drinking.
- Long-term alcohol abuse can turn into alcohol dependence.

Dependency on alcohol, also known as alcohol addiction and alcoholism,[1] is a chronic disease. The signs and symptoms of alcohol dependence include:

- A strong craving for alcohol.
- Continued use despite repeated physical, psychological, or interpersonal problems.
- The inability to limit drinking.

What is binge drinking?

According to the National Institute on Alcohol Abuse and Alcoholism binge drinking is defined as a pattern of alcohol consumption that brings the blood alcohol concentration (BAC) level to 0.08% or more. This pattern of drinking usually corresponds to 5 or more drinks on a single occasion for men or 4 or more drinks on a single occasion for women, generally within about 2 hours.

How do I know if it's okay to drink?

The current *Dietary Guidelines for Americans*[2] recommend that if you choose to drink alcoholic beverages you should not exceed 1 drink per day for women or 2 drinks per day for men. According to the guidelines, people who should not drink alcoholic beverages at all include the following:

- Children and adolescents.
- Individuals of any age who cannot limit their drinking to low level.
- Women who may become pregnant or who are pregnant.
- Individuals who plan to drive, operate machinery, or take part in other activities that require attention, skill, or coordination.
- Individuals taking prescription or over-the-counter medications that can interact with alcohol.
- Individuals with certain medical conditions.
- Persons recovering from alcoholism.

According to the *Dietary Guidelines for Americans*, it is not recommended that anyone begin drinking or drink more frequently on the basis of potential health benefits because moderate alcohol intake also is associated with increased risk of breast cancer, violence, drowning, and injuries from falls and motor vehicle crashes.

How do I know if I have a drinking problem?

Drinking is a problem if it causes trouble in your relationships, at school, with social activities, or in how you think and feel. If you are concerned that either you or someone in your family might have a drinking problem, consult your personal health-care provider.

Excessive drinking refers to per-occasion consumption or average consumption of alcohol that puts individuals at increased risk for alcohol-related health and social problems.[1] Excessive alcohol consumption is the third leading "actual" cause of death in the United States.[2]

Identifying My Developmental Tasks Homework

Review the age ranges and *circle* the tasks you are currently facing. It is common for individuals with chronic conditions to have developmental tasks from multiple ranges.

Ages and developmental tasks

(Ages 18–30) young adulthood
Selecting a mate. Learning to live with a partner. Starting family. Rearing children. Managing home. Getting started in occupation. Taking on civic responsibility. Finding a congenial social group.

At this stage of development, individuals are presented with tasks that focus on connecting with others by finding a partner and raising a family, finding a group of individuals to connect with for social outlets and support, connecting to one's community, and creating a stable living situation.

(Ages 30–60) middle age
Assisting teenage children to become responsible and happy adults. Achieving adult social and civic responsibility. Reaching and maintaining satisfactory performance in one's occupational career. Developing adult leisure-time activities. Relating oneself to one's spouse as a person. Accepting and adjusting to the physiological changes of middle age. Adjusting to aging parents.

At this stage of development, individuals are presented with the tasks of raising their children, building and maintaining a career, balancing work with healthy leisure activities, continuing to build intimacy with a partner, adjusting to how the body is changing with age, and coping with parents who are facing end-of-life issues.

(60 and over) older adulthood
Adjusting to decreasing physical strength and health. Adjusting to retirement and reduced income. Adjusting to death of a spouse. Establishing an explicit affiliation with one's age group. Adopting and adapting social roles in a flexible way. Establishing satisfactory physical living arrangements.

At this stage of development, individuals are presented with the tasks of adjusting to changes in their health and physical abilities, anticipating and planning for retirement, adjusting to changes in income, connecting with others who are in similar situations, changing social contacts and roles, and modifying or finding an appropriate place to live.

Lifespan Issues   NAME:_____
PSY

Working toward Healthy Development Homework

What is the developmental task you need to focus on?
(What is the task and from which stage)

_____

_____

_____

_____

Why is this currently a priority in your life?
(Want or need, for self or others, or both)

_____

_____

_____

_____

What do you hope to gain by working on this task?
(Emotional, financial, relationships)

_____

_____

_____

_____

What are your current resources and supports that can assist you?
(List your strengths and things/people that can help you)

_____

_____

_____

_____

What are your current barriers to accessing your resources and supports?
(What is getting in the way now and potentially in the future)

_____

_____

_____

_____

How can you begin working on this, what skills can you use, and what is the timeline?
(Commit to your plan)

_____

_____

_____

_____

Managing Flare-Ups   NAME: _____
PSY

Turning Fear and Inactivity into Action and Hope Homework

Past Activity _____

_____

Impact on Pain _____

_____

Lesson Learned _____

_____

How Reinforced _____

_____

Potential New Situation _____

_____

   How similar to old situation _____

   How different from old behavior _____

New Response + Lesson Learned _____

_____

New Message to Self – Cheerleading _____

_____

Possible Outcomes _____

_____

Action Strategies _____

_____

Disengagement Strategies _____

_____

Act – (Commitment) _____

_____

NAME: _____

Managing Conflict Homework

Have the individual develop a proactive action plan to incorporate MAD skills to use in times of conflict.

The skill set of **MAD (M)** is designed to manage conflict as it occurs. This skill set is similar to taking a time-out and interrupts the process of intense conflict.

Minimize – Acknowledge that conflict is occurring and minimize the chances of acting from a state of anger. Go to a different room or location, let the other person know when you will return to continue working on the issue, and find ways to "cool off."

Assess – Identify the level of your emotional distress and the intensity of the engagement. Prioritize the skills of DM, G, and F. Create a plan to re-engage when you and the other person are *both* ready to continue. If the situation is still intense, repeat the first skill until a safe and productive conversation can occur.

Damage control – Do not engage in hurtful words or actions. Do not allow yourself to be hurt or treated in a disrespectful manner. Repeat the two previous skills as needed.

Before the situation _____

_____

_____

_____

_____

During the situation _____

_____

_____

_____

_____

After the situation _____

_____

_____

_____

_____

The 3 Is   NAME: _____
SOC

The 3 Is Homework

Identity, insecurity, isolation

What is the issue you need to focus on?
(Identify and define the challenge)

_____

_____

_____

_____

Why is this currently a challenge in your life?
(Want or need, for self or others, or both)

_____

_____

_____

_____

What do you hope to gain by working on this challenge?
(Emotional, financial, relationships, stability)

_____

_____

_____

_____

What are your current resources and supports that can assist you?
(List your strengths and things/people that can help you)

_____

_____

_____

_____

What are your current barriers to accessing your resources and supports?
(What is getting in the way now and potentially in the future?)

_____

_____

_____

_____

How can you begin working on this, what skills can you use, and what is the timeline?
(Commit to your plan)

_____

_____

_____

_____

Individual-Based Problem-Solving Model Homework

The first strategy is for the individual who is addressing a problem without the involvement of others. This is done in a series of steps, and some steps may need to be repeated and modified throughout the process.

1. Identify the problem _____

    a. How is this impacting your thoughts, feelings and behaviors?

    _____

    _____

    _____

    _____

2. Review your values: _____

    a. Include your strengths and limitations:

    _____

    _____

    _____

    _____

    b. This includes yourself, others, and your environment (systems you are involved with):

    _____

    _____

    _____

    _____

3. Brainstorm potential solutions: _____

    a. No possibility is thrown out:

    _____

    _____

    _____

    _____

4. Consider the potential consequences of each decision: _____

    a. Narrow the possibilities and attach potential positive and negative conse-
        quences to each idea

    _____

    _____

    _____

    _____

    b. Create a pros and cons list for each potential solution

    _____

    _____

    _____

    _____

5. Select and implement the desired course of action: _____

    a. Evaluate whether the plan is working and needs to be continued, or whether
        it is not working as planned and needs to be modified or stopped

    _____

    _____

    _____

    _____

Problem-Solving   NAME: _____
SOC

Social-Based Problem-Solving Model

The second strategy is for the individual who is addressing a problem with the involvement of others. This is done in a series of steps, and some may need to be repeated and modified throughout the process.

1. Recognize the problem

    a. What is the problem? _____

       _____

       _____

    b. Why is it a problem? _____

       _____

       _____

    c. Who is involved now and potentially in the future? _____

       _____

       _____

2. Define the problem

    a. Create your own definition _____

       _____

       _____

    b. Consider factors of age, race, gender, values, and power differentials

       _____

       _____

    c. Get information and perspectives from others _____

       _____

       _____

3. Generate potential solutions

   a. Brainstorm potential solutions _____

   _____

   _____

   b. Create a pros and cons list for each potential solution _____

   _____

   _____

4. Select a potential solution _____

   _____

   _____

   a. Consider if the solution meets short-term, mid-term, or long-term needs

   _____

   _____

5. Review the process

   a. How did I reach this solution? _____

   _____

   _____

   b. Is the "golden rule" involved? _____

   _____

   c. Did I consider all of the relevant factors? _____

   _____

   _____

d. What is my motivation for this decision? _____

_____

_____

6. Implement and evaluate the solution _____

_____

_____

   a. Is new information available? _____

_____

   b. Do I need to continue, modify, or stop the plan? _____

_____

_____

_____

7. Reflect on the process

   a. What was learned? _____

_____

_____

_____

   b. How does this affect others, my environment, and me in the future?_____

_____

_____

_____

_____

Barriers to Nurturing Support Systems

There are many barriers to nurturing support systems. This list identifies many common examples and the potential hidden messages attached to each.

I am too busy (You are not worth the effort).

    Validation statement _____

    Challenge statement _____

I never thought of it (I don't consider your needs, I am too focused on myself).

    Validation statement _____

    Challenge statement _____

They don't want anything from me (I am not worthy of them).

    Validation statement _____

    Challenge statement _____

We fight all the time (It is too much of a bother to do/passive-aggressive).

    Validation statement _____

    Challenge statement _____

Our relationship never needed this before (I want things to be like they were).

    Validation statement _____

    Challenge statement _____

I am in too much pain or distress to do this now (It's not worth the effort).

    Validation statement _____

    Challenge statement _____

I can't (I don't know how).

Validation statement _____

Challenge statement _____

I won't (I can do this by myself).

Validation statement _____

Challenge statement _____

I don't know how (It is easier to avoid than to learn).

Validation statement _____

Challenge statement _____

When do I do something for them (It's not convenient for me)?

Validation statement _____

Challenge statement _____

I don't have money to spend on them (I can only show caring by buying gifts).

Validation statement _____

Challenge statement _____

I just want to be left alone (Let me suffer).

Validation statement _____

Challenge statement _____

Things are just fine the way that they are now (Denying reality).

Validation statement _____

Challenge statement _____

Social Roles
SOC

NAME: _____

Social Roles in Relationships

What is the issue you need to focus on?
(Defining a social role/social role transition)

_____

_____

_____

_____

Why is this currently a challenge in your life?
(Want or need, for self or others, or both)

_____

_____

_____

_____

What do you hope to gain by working on this challenge?
(Emotional, financial, relationships, stability)

_____

_____

_____

_____

What are your current resources and supports that can assist you?
(List your strengths and things/people that can help you)

_____

_____

_____

_____

What are your current barriers to accessing your resources and supports?
(What is getting in the way now and potentially in the future?)

How can you begin working on this, what skills can you use, and what is the timeline?
(Commit to your plan)

NAME: _____

Intimacy in Relationships

How do you define intimacy in your relationships?

_____

_____

_____

_____

What actions do you do to promote intimacy?

_____

_____

_____

_____

What actions would you like to engage in more often?

_____

_____

_____

_____

How do you anticipate others reacting?

_____

_____

_____

_____

How will this affect your relationships?

_____

_____

_____

_____

What is your plan to promote intimacy?

_____

_____

_____

_____

How will you know if your plan is working (review problem-solving models)?

_____

_____

_____

_____

Commit to your plan!

_____

_____

_____

_____

Styles of Interacting Handout

- **Personalizing** – An individual who over-identifies with the presented information and perceives that others are talking about them or that they are to blame for something.
    - *Need being met* – The individual feels connected to others and involved in the interaction.
    - *Potential social barrier* – Others may be annoyed by the individual making a situation be about themselves when that is not accurate. It can be a way to dominate conversations.
- **Fixing** – An individual who typically provides solutions to other people's problems even when solutions have not been requested.
    - *Need being met* – The individual feels valued and productive by helping to fix a problem.
    - *Potential social barrier* – Others may view the individual as being invalidating or feeling superior because the solutions are unsolicited.
- **Cheerleading** – An individual who encourages others by being overly optimistic and attempts to provide motivation to others in an unwavering manner.
    - *Need being met* – An individual feels supportive, helpful, and connected to others.
    - *Potential social barrier* – Others may view the individual's attempts to connect as being unhelpful, pushy, and overly optimistic.
- **Invalidating** – An individual who fails to connect to another person's experience and challenges or argues about what they "should" be experiencing.
    - *Need being met* – An individual is attempting to clarify what is happening so they can connect with others.
    - *Potential social barrier* – Others may feel hurt or misunderstood, causing them to disengage or withdraw.
- **Joining** – An individual who connects with other people through their pain or distress.
    - *Need being met* – An individual is attempting to connect with others by sharing their experiences with a similar problem.
    - *Potential social barrier* – Others may feel that the only topics for discussion center on pain and distress.
- **Tangential** – An individual who responds to others by connecting to minimally relevant aspects of the process or content of the interaction.
    - *Need being met* – An individual is attempting to either connect with others, or change the topic of discussion.
    - *Potential social barrier* – Others may perceive the individual as not following the conversation or as being uninterested.
- **Competition** – An individual who challenges others by competing with their stories and identifying with being better or worse than others in some aspect of their disclosures.

- ○ *Need being met* – An individual can relate to aspects of the conversation and wants to relate their story to others' stories.
- ○ *Potential social barrier* – Others may feel offended or devalued.
- **Masking** – An individual who hides or disguises their true experience and typically provides information that is not accurate to their own experience.
  - ○ *Need being met* – An individual is attempting to appear competent and confident so they are not perceived as being vulnerable.
  - ○ *Potential social barrier* – Others are not able to connect in a genuine manner.
- **Performing** – An individual who agrees with all feedback and challenges on a superficial level, and then either rejects change or attributes positives/blame to others.
  - ○ *Need being met* – An individual is able to deflect the focus of attention and avoid real or meaningful change.
  - ○ *Potential social barrier* – Others perceive the individual as being stubborn or resistant when "old behaviors or patterns" return once the pressure to conform is removed.
- **Externalizing** – An individual attributes credit for success or failure to others in a consistent manner.
  - ○ *Need being met* – An individual is able to give others compliments or deflect responsibility and blame onto others.
  - ○ *Potential social barrier* – Others may feel angry, blamed, or disrespected.
- **Help-rejecting complaining** – An individual identifies a problem and then dismisses all potential solutions.
  - ○ *Need being met* – An individual is able to avoid changing or "being fixed" by others.
  - ○ *Potential social barrier* – Others may perceive the individual as whining and not wanting the help and support that they are offering.
- **Finding extremes** – An individual uses extremes in language, thoughts, or behaviors.
  - ○ *Need being met* – An individual is attempting to clarify and simplify their experience by deleting the complexity of the situation or experience.
  - ○ *Potential social barrier* – Others cannot connect with a "middle ground" or common experience.

Styles of Interacting   NAME: _____
SOC

Styles of Interacting Homework

Personalizing – An individual who over-identifies with the presented information and perceives that others are talking about them or that they are to blame for something.

- Need being met – _____

- Potential social barrier – _____

- Alternative action strategy – _____

Fixing – An individual who typically provides solutions to other people's problems even when solutions have not been requested.

- Need being met – _____

- Potential social barrier – _____

- Alternative action strategy – _____

Cheerleading – An individual who encourages others by being overly optimistic and attempts to provide motivation to others in an unwavering manner.

- Need being met – _____

- Potential social barrier – _____

- Alternative action strategy – _____

Invalidating – An individual who fails to connect to another person's experience and challenges or argues about what they "should" be experiencing.

- Need being met – _____

- Potential social barrier – _____

- Alternative action strategy – _____

Joining – An individual who connects with other people through their pain or distress.

- ○ Need being met – _____

- ○ Potential social barrier – _____

- ○ Alternative action strategy – _____

Tangential – An individual who responds to others by connecting to minimally relevant aspects of the process or content of the interaction.

- ○ Need being met – _____

- ○ Potential social barrier – _____

- ○ Alternative action strategy – _____

Competition – An individual who challenges others by competing with their stories and identifying with being better or worse than others in some aspect of their disclosures.

- ○ Need being met – _____

- ○ Potential social barrier – _____

- ○ Alternative action strategy – _____

Masking – An individual who hides or disguises their true experience and typically provides information that is not accurate to their own experience.

- ○ Need being met – _____

- ○ Potential social barrier – _____

- ○ Alternative action strategy – _____

Performing – An individual who agrees with all feedback and challenges on a superficial level, and then either rejects change or attributes positives/blame to others.

- ○ Need being met – _____

- ○ Potential social barrier – _____

- ○ Alternative action strategy – _____

Externalizing – An individual attributes credit for success or failure to others in a consistent manner.

- ○ Need being met – _____

- ○ Potential social barrier – _____

- ○ Alternative action strategy – _____

Help-rejecting complaining – An individual identifies a problem and then dismisses all potential solutions.

- ○ Need being met – _____

- ○ Potential social barrier – _____

- ○ Alternative action strategy – _____

Finding extremes – An individual uses extremes in language, thoughts, or behaviors.

- ○ Need being met – _____

- ○ Potential social barrier – _____

- ○ Alternative action strategy – _____

Master Skills Sheet

BIO

Session: Goal setting and motivation

Observe (OBS) – Noticing one's experience

Describe (DES) – The process of putting words on one's experience

Participate (PART) – Noting what the individual doing to cope with the current situation and how present they are in the process

Non-Judgmental Stance (NJS) – Noticing our experience without placing value on the experience itself or the process

One-Mindfully (OM) – Focusing our attention on the present situation or task

Effectively (EFF) – Doing what is required to meet needs in a healthy manner

Radical Acceptance (RA). This skill may be defined as accepting reality for what it is.

Practical Acceptance (PA). This skill may be defined as accepting reality and understanding that controlling the situation is futile, but that the individual can still influence the situation.

Practical Change (PC). This skill may be defined as changing many aspects of a situation and needing to accept some aspects that are change resistant.

Radical Change (RC). This skill may be defined as changing all aspects of a situation because no other alternatives are acceptable.

Session: Functioning and loss

Behavioral Mapping – The individual is to track their activities throughout the day, how they attempted to cope, levels of pain pre/post intervention, and the location or source of their pain.

CBT for Chronic Pain and Psychological Well-Being: A Skills Training Manual Integrating DBT, ACT, Behavioral Activation and Motivational Interviewing, First Edition. Mark Carlson.
© 2014 John Wiley & Sons, Ltd. Published 2014 by John Wiley & Sons, Ltd.

Event Scheduling – The individual is to complete the plan early in treatment and modify the plan as they learn and apply coping skills throughout the course of the program.

Modifying Activities – Review frequency (F) of the activity, intensity (I) of engagement, and duration (D) of involvement and altering aspects of FID through attempts at self-regulation and pacing strategies.

Building Mastery (BM) – Engaging in activities that have a high probability of success.

Building Positive Experiences (BPE) – Engaging in activities that improve quality of life through the individual experiencing a heightened sense of positive emotions.

Mood Momentum (MM) – Noticing and engaging in positive experiences and selecting skills to stay engaged in the activity.

Session: sleep

Building a Routine – Go to bed when you are sleepy; do not force your sleep; set a consistent time to start your bed-time ritual that assists in preparing you for sleep; if you do not fall asleep after 20 minutes, you need to get out of bed; find a distraction that does not involve strenuous activity and is short in duration; when you become sleepy go back to bed; get out of bed at the same time every morning; establish a bedtime ritual that helps you prepare for sleep; engage in activities that calm the mind and body; keep your bedroom cool, quiet, and dark; keep to your schedule; avoid naps if at all possible.

Maintaining a Routine – Bed is for sleep so minimize other activities done in your bed; minimize or stop caffeine intake after mid-afternoon; avoid any alcohol consumption within 6 hours of bedtime; avoid big meals or being too hungry before bedtime; avoid exercising 6 hours before bedtime; have a plan to cope with worry thoughts; list strategies to get back to sleep; consult your doctor.

Session: Adherence to treatment protocols

DEAR MAN (DM) is designed to teach the individual to increase the probability of getting their wants or needs met.

Describe – Use Observe and Describe to summarize the situation and identify the facts that support the request or reason for setting a limit or boundary.

Express – Share your beliefs or opinions when relevant or required.

Assert – Ask clearly for what you want or need.

Reward – Let others know how helping you meet your wants or needs will potentially impact their situation.

Mindful – Stay focused on your request and avoid leaving the topic.

Act confident – Use an assertive tone, have confident body language, make eye contact, and stay calm.

Negotiate – Be willing to compromise to meet your wants or needs.

GIVE (G) is designed to teach the individual to build and maintain relationships.

Gentle – Be respectful in your approach and avoid threats, demands, and attacks.

Interested – Listen to the other person and be open to the information they have to provide.

Validate – Acknowledge and attempt to understand the other person's perspective.

Easy Manner – Be political and treat others in a kind and relaxed manner.

FAST (F) is designed to teach the individual how to have self-respect and self-worth.

Fair – Be fair to yourself and others.

Apologies – Do not engage in unnecessary apologetic behavior.

Stick to values – Use your own value system as a guide for your behavior.

Truthful – Be honest and accountable to yourself and others.

Session: Complexity

Validation (V) – To acknowledge, confirm, authenticate, verify, or prove. This concept may be simple to understand, but is very difficult to apply in a consistent and effective manner to ourselves.

Session: Working with your team

Preparing for appointments – Prioritize needs and wants; set clear goals and objectives for the appointment; create a list of questions for the professional; organize the tracking forms and tracking cards; plan for childcare if needed; plan or coordinate transportation; plan for an advocate to attend if needed; visualize the appointment.

Structuring the day of the appointment can assist in this process as well.

KEEP IT REAL – **K**ey in on the task at hand, be respectful and take an active role in your care; **e**stablish the goals and objectives, provide information, make consistent "I" statements and take responsibility for your decisions and care; **t**ake notes; **r**equest written materials; **a**sk questions, be assertive; **e**ngage in reflective communication; **l**eave with a clear care plan, know what the next steps in your care are and discuss them with the professional before leaving.

Grounding Yourself (GY) – Grounding exercises bring you back to the here and now.

Willingness (W) – Meeting others and situations where they are at instead of where we wish they were.

Non-judgmental Stance (NJS) – Understanding when to use judgments and when to let them go.

PSY

Session: Depression

Safety – The first priority is to assess for safety in all individuals. If the individual is experiencing suicidal ideation this must be addressed before any other issues. A clear commitment to safety is a primary requirement for continued therapy.

Building Positive Experiences (BPE) – Creating or engaging in activities that lead to positive moods.

Just Noticeable Change (JNC) – Engaging in a behavior the leads to a change in focus or direction.

Session: Anxiety

Distracting the mind – Engaging in activities that disrupt current thought patterns.

Imagery – Picturing (in your mind's eye) yourself tolerating the distress.

Soothing through the senses – Engaging the five senses to promote a sense of peace and serenity.

PLEASED (PL) – Self-care skills promote well-being and reduce emotional vulnerability.

   Physical Health – Taking medicines as prescribed, following medical protocols, and making appointments (and attending them) when necessary.

   List resources and barriers – Create a list of strengths and resources for each area of this skill. Create a list of barriers for potential problem-solving in session.

   Eat balanced meals – Eat three balanced meals plus healthy snacks throughout the day.

   Avoid drugs and alcohol – There are many risks associated with using drugs and alcohol.

   Sleep – Healthy sleep is a must!

   Exercise – Exercise a minimum of 20 minutes three to five times weekly.

   Daily – Practice these skills every day to create healthy habits.

Session: Attending to distress

Distract with ACCEPTS – Accept distress to effectively apply distraction skills.

   Activities – Activities assist in decreasing distress and can create positive emotions. Plan activities and do something each day. Doing something is often better than doing nothing. Create an activities list of things you enjoy doing to promote a more active and healthy approach to coping with distress.

   Contributing – Do something for someone else. Take a break from your own distress by engaging in others' lives in a positive manner. Smiling, volunteering support or assistance, and listening are all examples of this skill.

   Comparisons – Compare your current situation to a time where you were less skillful and less effective. This can provide perspective to your current situation. You can also compare your situation to that of someone who has it worse than you. Validate your experience as you search for healthy perspectives.

Emotions – Engage in activities or thoughts that create emotions that are different from the painful ones you are currently experiencing.

Push Away – Mentally put the distress in a box on a shelf behind a locked door. Take a break from it now with the intention of addressing the issue at a safe point in the future.

Thoughts – Engage in activities that lead to different thoughts. Read a book or magazine, work a puzzle, or count to 100.

Sensations – Stimulate sensations that are safe to engage in.

Turning the Mind (TTM) – Continually refocusing your attention and concentration away from the distress to the distraction activity. This may need to be done continually to be effective.

Session: Stigma

Thought-Stopping – Say "STOP" when you experience automatic negative thoughts (ANTS).

Positive Self-Talk – Replace negative messages and "old tapes that play in your head" with positive messages by creating "new tapes" that you create.

Session: Chemical abuse

Urge Surfing (US) – Accepting distressing urges and emotions and riding the ups and downs of the experience like a surfer rides a wave.

Bridge Burning (BB) – Removing the means to act on potentially harmful urges.

SOC

Session: Managing conflict

MAD (M) – is designed to manage conflict as it occurs. This skill set is similar to taking a time-out and interrupts the process of intense conflict.

Minimize – Acknowledge that conflict is occurring and minimize the chances of acting from a state of anger.

Assess – Identify the level of your emotional distress and the intensity of the engagement.

Damage control – Do not engage in hurtful words or actions.

Session: Identity/isolation/insecurity

Wise Mind (WM) can be used to find balance between feelings of security and insecurity.

Opposite to Emotion (O2E) – Use opposite actions to avoid negative emotions.

Master Skills Reference List

BIO

Session: Goal Setting and Motivation
   Observe (OBS) (Linehan, 1993b)
   Describe (DES) (Linehan, 1993b)
   Participate (PART) (Linehan, 1993b)
   Non-judgmental Stance (NJS) (Linehan, 1993b)
   One-Mindfully (OM) (Linehan, 1993b)
   Effective (EFF) (Linehan, 1993b)
   Radical Acceptance (RA) (Linehan, 1993b)
   Practical Acceptance (PA) (Carlson, 2014 (*the current volume*))
   Practical Change (PC) (Carlson, 2014)
   Radical Change (RC) (Linehan, 1993b)
Session: Functioning and Loss
   Behavioral Mapping
   Event Scheduling
   Modifying Activities
   Building Mastery (BM) (Linehan, 1993b)
   Building Positive Experiences (BPE) (Carlson, 2014)
   Mood Momentum (MM) (Pederson & Pederson, 2012)
Session: Sleep
   Building a routine (Pederson & Pederson, 2012)
   Maintaining a routine (Pederson & Pederson, 2012)
Session: Adherence to Treatment Protocols
   Dear Man (DM) (Linehan, 1993b)
   Give (G) (Linehan, 1993b)
   Fast (F) (Linehan, 1993b)
Session: Complexity
   Validation (V) (Linehan, 1993b and Pederson & Pederson, 2012)
Session: Working with Your Team
   Preparing for an appointment (Carlson, 2014)
   KEEP IT REAL (Carlson, 2014)
   Ground Yourself (GY) (Pederson & Pederson, 2012)
   Willingness (W) (Linehan, 1993b)

PSY

Session: Depression
   Safety
   Building Positive Experiences (BPE) (Linehan, 1993b)
   Just Noticeable Change (JNC) (Carlson, 2014)
Session: Anxiety
   Distracting the Mind (Linehan, 1993b)
   Imagery (Linehan, 1993b)

Soothing through the Senses (Linehan, 1993b)
PLEASED (PL) (Linehan, 1993b)
Session: Attending to Distress
Distract with ACCEPTS (Linehan, 1993b)
Turning the Mind (TTM) (Linehan, 1993b)
Session: Stigma
Thought-Stopping through Positive Self-Talk
Session: Chemical Abuse
Urge Surfing (US) (Pederson & Pederson, 2012)
Bridge Burning (BB) (Linehan, Unpublished) (Pederson & Pederson, 2012)

SOC

Session: Managing Conflict
MAD (M) (Carlson, 2014)
Session: Identity/Isolation/Insecurity
Wise Mind (WM) (Linehan, 1993b)
Opposite to Emotion (O2E) (Linehan, 1993b)

Appendix

Safety Contract

I, _____, contract for my safety. This means I will not act on any plan to commit suicide. I will use my skills to assist with my safety, call my team members/people in my support system/crisis numbers as needed, or admit myself into the hospital if needed.

As a part of my safety contract, I will also attend all scheduled appointments and my group. Not attending group or other appointments as planned will be considered a violation of my willingness to commit to safety.

Client signature and date: _____

Therapist signature and date: _____

Original to client; copy to chart

CBT for Chronic Pain and Psychological Well-Being: A Skills Training Manual Integrating DBT, ACT, Behavioral Activation and Motivational Interviewing, First Edition. Mark Carlson.
© 2014 John Wiley & Sons, Ltd. Published 2014 by John Wiley & Sons, Ltd.

References

(Chapter numbers and sections in brackets refer to the current volume)

American Academy of Pain Medicine. (n.d.). AAPM facts and figures on pain. Retrieved April 2012 from http://www.painmed.org/PatientCenter/Facts_on_Pain.aspx.

American Psychiatric Association. (2000). *Diagnostic and statistical manual of mental disorders* (Revised 4th ed.). Washington, DC.

American Psychological Association. (2010, November 9). Stress in America findings. Retrieved April 2012 from http://www.stressinamerica.org.

American Society of Anesthesiologists. (2010). Practice guidelines for chronic pain management. *Anesthesiology, 112*(4): 1–24.

Arkowitz, H. (1992) Integrative theories of therapy. In D. K. Freedheim (ed.). *History of psychotherapy: A century of change*, pp. 261–303). Washington, DC: American Psychological Association (Chapter 2).

Bosworth, H. (ed.). (2010). *Improving patient treatment adherence: A clinician's guide*. Breinigsville, PA: Springer.

Brody, T. A. (1993). *The philosophy behind physics*. Edited by L. De La Pena and P. E. Hodgson. Berlin, Germany: Springer Verlag.

Burrows, B. (2006, September 11). How stress works. Retrieved from http://science.howstuffworks.com/environmental/life/human-biology/how-stress-works.htm.

Centers for Disease Control and Prevention. (2011). Retrieved March 1, 2012 from http://www.cdc.gov/chronicdisease/overview/index.htm.

Committee on Advancing Pain Research, Care, and Education, & Institute of Medicine. (2011, June 29). Relieving pain in America: A blueprint for transforming prevention, care, education, and research. Retrieved April 2012 from http://http://iom.edu/~/media/Files/Report%20Files/2011/Relieving-Pain-in-America-A-Blueprint-for-Transforming-Prevention-Care-Education-Research/Pain%20Research%202011%20Report%20Brief.pdf

Elliott, A. M., Smith B. H., Penny K. I., Smith W. C., & Chambers W. A. (1999). The epidemiology of chronic pain in the community. *Lancet, 354*(9186): 1248–1252.

Engel, G. L. (1977). The need for a new medical model: A challenge for biomedicine. *Science, 196*: 129–136. (Chapter 2).

Evans, D. R., Burns, J. E., Robinson, W. E., & Garrett, O. J. (1985). The quality of life questionnaire: A multidimensional measure. *American Journal of Community Psychology, 13*: 305–322. (Chapter 2).

Fishbain, D. A., Rosomoff, H. L., & Rosomoff, R. S. (1992). Drug abuse, dependence, and addiction in chronic pain patients. *The Clinical Journal of Pain, 8*: 77–85.

Frank, J. D., & Frank, J. B. (1991). *Persuasion and healing* (3rd ed.). Baltimore, MD: John Hopkins University Press. (Chapter 2).

Gatchel, R .J. (2004). Comorbidity of chronic pain and mental health disorders: The biopsychosocial perspective. *American Psychologist, 59*(8): 795–805.

Gatchel, R. J., Peng, Y. B., Peters, M. L., Fuchs, P. N., & Turk, D. C. (2007). The biopsychosocial approach to chronic pain: Scientific advances and future directions. *Psychological Bulletin, 133*(4): 581–624.

Glenn, B., & Burns, J. W. (2003). Pain self-management in the process and outcome of multidisciplinary treatment of chronic pain: Evaluation of a stage change model. *Journal of Behavioral Medicine, 26*(5): 417–433.

Green, C., Wheeler, J., Marchant, B., LaPorte, F., & Guerrero, E. (2011). Analysis of the physician variable in pain management. *Pain Medicine, 2*(4): 317–327.

Gottman, J. M., & Levenson, R. W. (1992). Marital processes predictive of later dissolution: Behavior, physiology, and health. *Journal of Personality and Social Psychology, 63*: 221–233. (Chapter 3, Psychological Curriculum: Anger Management session).

Havighurst, R. J. (1972). *Developmental tasks and education* (3rd ed.). New York: NY. Longman.

Hayes, S. C., Hayes, L. J., & Reese, H. W. (1988). Finding the philosophical core [Review of the book World hypotheses: A study in evidence, by S. C. Pepper]. *Journal of the Experimental Analysis of Behavior, 50*: 97–111.

Hill, M., Glaser, K., & Harden, J. (1998). A feminist model for ethical decision making. *Women & Therapy, 21*(3): 101–121.

Holtberg, B. (2013). Unpublished script for a guided imagery technique.

Kabat-Zinn, J. (1991). *Full catastrophe living*. New York, NY: Dell Publishing.

Kelley, H. H. (1973). The processes of causal attribution. *American psychologist, 28*(2): 107–128.

Kerns, R. D., Rosenberg, R., Jamison, R. N., Caudill, M. A., & Haythornthwaite, J. (1997). Readiness to adopt a self-management approach to chronic pain: The pain stages of change questionnaire (PSOCQ). *Pain, 72*: 227–234. (Chapter 3, Psychological Curriculum: Readiness to Change session).

Kirsh, K. L. (2010). Differentiating and managing common psychiatric comorbidities seen in chronic pain patients. *Journal of Pain & Palliative Care Pharmacotherapy, 24*(1): 39–47.

Kraus, D. R., Seligman, D. A., & Jordan, J. R. (2005). Validation of a behavioral health treatment outcome and assessment tool designed for naturalistic settings: The treatment outcome package. *Journal of Clinical Psychology, 61*(3): 285–314. (Chapter 2).

Lemay, R. A. (1999). Roles, identities, and expectancies: Positive contributions to normalization and social role volarization. In R. J. Flynn and R. A. Lemay (eds). *A quarter-century of normalization and social role volarization: Evolution and Impact*. Ottawa, ON: University of Ottawa Press.

Lewandowski, M. J. (2006). *The chronic pain care workbook: A self-treatment approach to pain relief using the behavioral assessment of pain questionnaire*. Oakland, CA: New Harbinger Publications, Inc.

Linehan, M. M. (1993a). *Cognitive-behavioral treatment of borderline personality disorder*. New York, NY: The Guilford Press.

Linehan, M. M. (1993b). *Skills training manual for treating borderline personality disorder.* New York, NY: The Guilford Press.

Linton, S. J., & Nordin. E. (2006). A five-year follow-up evaluation of the health and economic consequences of an early cognitive-behavioral intervention for back pain: A randomized, controlled trial. *Spine, 31*: 853–858.

Lorig, K., Holman, H., Sobel, K., Laurent, D., Gonzalez, V., & Minor, M. (2006). *Living a healthy life with chronic conditions* (3rd ed.). Boulder, CO: Bull Publishing Company.

Martinez, Y. K. (2009). Chronic illnesses in Canadian children: What is the effect of illness on academic achievement, and anxiety and emotional disorders? *Child: Care, Health & Development, 35*(3): 391–401.

Melzack, R., & Wall, P. D. (1988). *The challenge of pain.* New York, NY: Penguin Books. (Chapter 2).

Morely, S., Eccleston, C., & Williams, A. (1999). Systemic review and meta-analysis of randomized controlled trials of cognitive behavior therapy and behavior therapy for chronic pain in adults, excluding headache. *Pain, 80*: 1–13.

Novaco, R. W. (1983). *Stress inoculation therapy for anger controls: A manual for therapists.* Unpublished manuscript, Irvine. (Chapter 3, Psychological Curriculum: Anger Management session).

Novaco, R. W. (1985). *Anger, stress, and coping with provocation: An instruction manual.* Unpublished manuscript, Irvine. (Chapter 3, Psychological Curriculum: Anger Management session).

Osburn, J. (2006). An overview of social role volarization theory. *The SRV Journal, 1*(1): 4–13.

Ownsworth, T. (2009). A biopsychosocial perspective on adjustment and quality of life following brain tumor: A systematic evaluation of the literature. *Disability & Rehabilitation, 31*(13): 1038–1055.

Pederson, L., & Pederson, C. S. (2012). *The expanded dialectical behavior therapy skills training manual.* Eau Claire, WI: Premier Publishing & Media.

Prochaska, J., & Velicer, W. (1997). The transtheoretical model of health behavior change. *American Journal of Health Promotion, 12*(1): 38–48.

Rotter, J. B. (1954). *Social learning and clinical psychology.* New York, NY: Prentice-Hall. (Chapter 3, Psychological Curriculum: Orientation to Change session).

Sharp, J., & Keefe, B. (2006). Psychiatry in chronic pain: A review and update. *Focus, 4*(4): 573–580.

Strang, P., Strang, S., Hultborn, R., & Arner, S. (2004). Existential pain – an entity, a provocation, or a challenge? *Journal of Pain and Symptom Management, 27*(3): 241–250. (Chapter 3, Psychological Curriculum: Meaning and Pain session).

Stuart, S. (2008). What is IPT? The basic principles and the inevitability of change. *Journal of Contemporary Psychotherapy, 38*: 1–10. Retrieved April 2013 from http://www.slideshare.net/sharonrafael/what-is-ipt-stuart-2008.

Thomas, S. and Wolfensberger, W. (1999). An overview of social role valorization. In Flynn, R. J. and Lemay, R. A. *A quarter century of normalization and social role valorization: Evolution and impact.* Ottawa: University of Ottawa Press.

Wampold, B. E. (2001). *The great psychotherapy debate: Models, methods, and findings.* Mahwah, NJ: Lawrence Erlbaum Associates. (Chapter 2).

Index

CBT for Chronic Pain and Psychological Well-Being: A Skills Training Manual Integrating DBT, ACT, Behavioral Activation and Motivational Interviewing, First Edition. Mark Carlson.
© 2014 John Wiley & Sons, Ltd. Published 2014 by John Wiley & Sons, Ltd.

Printed and bound by CPI Group (UK) Ltd, Croydon, CR0 4YY

27/10/2024

14580222-0001